Assisting in the Pharmacy

by Gail Askew, PharmD, FCSHP and
Marilyn Smith-Stoner, RN, MSN, PhD

Clinical Allied Healthcare Series

Kay Stevens, RN, MA
Series Editor

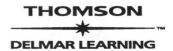

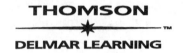

Assisting in the Pharmacy
by Gail Askew, PharmD, FCSHP and
Marilyn Smith-Stoner, RN, MSN, PhD

Senior Editor and Executive Director:
Kay Stevens

Senior Editor and Project Coordinator:
Valerie L. Harris

Editors:
William C. Klein
Karlene Miller
Beverly Marshburn
Jacquelyn R. Marshall

Production Artists:
William c. Klein
Karlene Miller
Valerie L. Harris

Illustrators:
William C. Klein
Alan J. Borie
Valerie L. Harris

Cover Design:
Harris Graphics

Additional Graphics obtained from the LifeART™ Collections from Lippincott Williams & Wilkins, Cleveland, OH

10 9 8 7 6 5 4
ISBN 0-89262-438-8
Library of Congress Catalog Card Number 00-108727

NOTICE TO THE READER

Publisher does not warrant or guarantee any of the products described herein or perform any independent analysis in connection with any of the product information contained herein. Publisher does not assume, and expressly disclaims, any obligation to obtain and include information other than that provided to it by the manufacturer.

The reader is expressly warned to consider and adopt all safety precautions that might be indicated by the activities herein and to avoid all potential hazards. By following the instructions contained herein, the reader willingly assumes all risks in connection with such instructions.

The Publisher makes no representation or warranties of any kind, including but not limited to, the warranties of fitness for particular purpose or merchantability, nor are any such representations implied with respect to the material set forth herein, and the publisher takes no responsibility with respect to such material. The publisher shall not be liable for any special, consequential, or exemplary damages resulting, in whole or part, from the readers' use of, or reliance upon, this material.

Contents

Acknowledgements vii

Introduction viii

Contributors ix

Editor's Note xii

Chapter One
Introduction to the Pharmacy 1-1
   Objectives 1-1
   Key Terms 1-2
   Introduction 1-2
   Assistants in the Pharmacy and Their Titles 1-3
   Characteristics of Pharmacy Personnel 1-4
   Responding to Customers with Care 1-6
   Technical Training 1-7
   Places of Employment 1-8
      The Hospital Environment 1-9
      The Outpatient Pharmacy 1-11
      Other Types of Pharmacies 1-12
   Professional Organizations 1-13
      Web Sites 1-13
   Chapter Summary 1-14
   Student Enrichment Activities 1-15

Chapter Two
The Pharmacy Team 2-1
   Objectives 2-1
   Key Terms 2-2
   Introduction 2-2
   The Pharmacist 2-2
   The Pharmacy Technician 2-5
   The Pharmacy Clerk 2-7
   The Prescriber 2-8
   The Business Manager 2-10
   Drug Suppliers and Salespeople 2-11
   Other Healthcare Workers 2-11
   The Organizational Structure of a Pharmacy 2-12
   Chapter Summary 2-14
   Student Enrichment Activities 2-15

Chapter Three
Essential Skills and Responsibilities 3-1
    Objectives 3-1
    Key Terms 3-2
    Introduction 3-2
    Customer Service 3-2
    Effective Communication 3-8
    Operating Business Machines in the Pharmacy 3-11
        The Cash Register 3-11
        The Credit Card Scanner 3-13
    Accepting a Check for Payment 3-16
    Insurance Plans and Drug Reimbursement 3-17
    Avoiding Cross-Contamination 3-26
        Contamination of Medications 3-29
        Needle Disposal 3-29
    Committee Assignments 3-30
    Chapter Summary 3-30
    Student Enrichment Activities 3-31

Chapter Four
Pharmacology Basics 4-1
    Objectives 4-1
    Key Terms 4-2
    Introduction 4-2
    Drugs and Their Development 4-2
    Drug Naming 4-4
        Drug Salts 4-5
        Slang Names 4-6
    Drug Classifications 4-6
        Controlled Substances 4-7
    Routes of Administration 4-9
    Drug Dosage Forms 4-10
        Oral Solids 4-10
        Oral Liquids 4-12
        Topical Dosage Forms 4-13
        Injectables 4-15
    Dosages 4-15
    Drug Effects 4-17
    Drug Reference Materials 4-18
    Pharmacologic Categories of Medication 4-21
        Antimicrobials (Anti-infectives) 4-21
        Antineoplastics 4-22

Contents

    Electrolyte Replacements 4-22
    Cardiovascular System Medications 4-23
    Digestive System Medications 4-25
    Endocrine (Hormone) System Medications 4-26
    Nervous System Medications 4-28
    Musculoskeletal System Medications 4-31
    Respiratory System Medications 4-31
    Urinary System Medications 4-32
Chapter Summary 4-33
Student Enrichment Activities 4-35

Chapter Five
The Prescription 5-1
Objectives 5-1
Key Terms 5-2
Introduction 5-2
The Elements of a Prescription 5-3
Prescription Processing – Part 1 5-4
Abbreviations 5-6
Measurements Used in the Pharmacy 5-7
Prescription Labels 5-11
Warning/Auxiliary Labels 5-12
Prescription Processing – Part 2 5-13
Taking Telephone Orders 5-14
Patient Confidentiality 5-15
Fraudulent Prescriptions 5-17
Pharmacy Theft 5-18
Chapter Summary 5-19
Student Enrichment Activities 5-21

Chapter Six
Inventory Control in the Pharmacy 6-1
Objectives 6-1
Key Terms 6-2
Introduction 6-2
Shelf Life 6-2
Purchasing 6-3
    Controlled Substances 6-4
Stocking Shelves 6-5
    Stocking Shelves in a Retail Pharmacy 6-6
    Stocking Shelves in the Hospital Pharmacy 6-8
    Stocking Shelves in the Home Infusion Pharmacy 6-10
Drug Distribution in a Hospital Pharmacy 6-10

    Unit Dose Distribution 6-12
    Automated Dispensing Systems 6-15
Transporting Medication 6-16
    Transporting Medication in a Hospital Pharmacy 6-16
    Transporting Medications from a Retail or Home
       Infusion Pharmacy 6-16
Chapter Summary 6-18
Student Enrichment Activities 6-19

Chapter Seven
Staying Healthy in the Workplace 7-1
Objectives 7-1
Key Terms 7-2
Introduction 7-2
Maintaining Good Health 7-2
    Control Your Weight 7-2
    Get Plenty of Exercise 7-6
    Get Plenty of Sleep 7-7
    Avoid Hypertension 7-7
    Manage Stress 7-7
    Avoid the Inappropriate Use of Alcohol and Drugs 7-8
Workplace Safety 7-9
    Biohazardous Substances in the Pharmacy 7-9
    Health Tips for Computer Users 7-9
    Preventing Sprains and Strains 7-10
    Avoiding Falls 7-11
    Robberies 7-11
Chapter Summary 7-11
Student Enrichment Activities 7-13

Appendix A
Glossary .... Appendix A-1

Appendix B
The Manual Alphabet .... Appendix B-1

Appendix C
Bibliography .... Appendix C-1

Appendix D
Index .... Appendix D-1

Acknowledgements

The authors would like to thank everyone who graciously contributed to the formation of this text. The contributions of the following are particularly appretciated.

Kay Stevens, RN, MA, Series Editor and Executive Director, for conceiving this series and for her valued assistance in making this book a reality.

Jim Brodsky, RPh, DHPh, ND, and the staff of Villa Park Pharmacy in Villa Park, California, for their kind assistance in helping us stage photographs and for providing helpful information on emerging trends in the pharmacy.

Karen Olen, RPh, for providing us with valuable pharmaceutical information.

Lawrence E. Woodhouse, PharmD, and the staff of Yorba Park Pharmacy in Orange, California, for their gracious assistance in helping us stage photographs.

Introduction

To work in the medical field is to make a real contribution to your fellow man. This is a career that will ask much of your mind and heart and give much in return. The satisfaction gained from calming a frightened child or brightening the day of a lonely patient will enrich you. The pride felt will be lasting when your observations and skills someday help to save a patient's life. This is a career where you can really make a difference!

Some of you have already made a decision to seek a career in some area of healthcare. Some of you are just exploring your options. Everything you learn will build a foundation of skills and knowledge, so learn well. Become competent in everything you are taught along the way and be your own task master. We all must be responsible for our own education. If at some point you discover you didn't learn a skill well enough, go back and practice until you do. Remember, some day a patient's life may depend on you and your mastery of what you are taught.

Today's healthcare industry places many demands on care givers. We must keep costs down, document everything we do, and have more knowledge and skills than ever before because of new technology. This textbook series was designed to help you build a sound foundation of knowledge and provide many opportunities for cross-training. The core textbook contains the skills and information we feel is common to all students. Each of the other textbooks provide training for a specific job title. The more you can learn, the better. Always remember, however, to practice the art, the science, and the SPIRIT of your new career. Good luck!

Kay Stevens, RN, MA
Series Editor

Contributors

About the Co-Authors
Gail Askew, PharmD, FCSHP, received her doctorate in pharmacy from the University of Southern California in 1974. Following graduation, Dr. Askew completed a pharmacy residency at the University of California, Irvine, Medical Center and began a career that has included acute care and community pharmacy practice, as well as healthcare education.

Dr. Askew has nearly 25 years of experience in pharmacy technician training. Currently, Dr. Askew serves as professor and chairperson of the Pharmacy Technology Department at Santa Ana College in Santa Ana, CA. Under her guidance, Santa Ana College became the first community college in the nation to receive accreditation from the American Society of Health-Systems Pharmacists (ASHP).

Dr. Askew has an extensive history of service to the pharmacy community. On the national level, Dr. Askew is a content expert on ASHP's accreditation site survey teams. She participated in the initial development of the Pharmacy Technician Certification Board (PTCB) exam. Additionally, Dr. Askew has served as a consultant in the development of numerous pharmacy technician training programs, including Project Hope's program in Pima County, AZ.

Dr. Askew is active in both state and local pharmacy organizations, having served two terms as the pharmacist member-at-large to the Technician Division of the California Society of Health-System Pharmacists (CSHP). Dr. Askew is a current member of the CSHP Council on Organizational Affairs and is a past president of the Orange County Society of Health-System Pharmacists. Dr. Askew was selected as an Outstanding Young Woman of America in 1986. In 1999, Dr. Askew was recognized for her contributions to the pharmacy profession by being named a Fellow of the California Society of Health-System Pharmacists.

Marilyn Smith-Stoner, RN, MSN, PhD received her Bachelor of Science degree in 1989 and Master of Science degree in 1995 from California State University, Dominguez Hills, California, and recently earned her Doctoral degree from California Institute of Integral Studies, in San Francisco, California. The focus of Dr. Smith-Stoner's research is meaningful learning in the on-line graduate classroom, which clearly complements her professional commitments as a Distance Learning Specialist at California State University, Fullerton; Vice President of Operations for the Ramona Visiting Nurses Association and Hospice, in Hemet, California; and Adjunct Professor to University of Phoenix, in Arizona, and Baker College On-line, in Michigan.

Early in her career, Dr. Smith-Stoner established herself as a dynamic force in the healthcare field, receiving the Outstanding Achievement Award: Governor's Employment of the Handicapped, in 1982, and being honored in association with the *1985 Who's Who on Young Women in America* and the *1986 Who's Who in American Nursing*. Over the intervening years, Dr. Smith-Stoner has been employed as a staff nurse at several southern California medical facilities and has taught a wide variety of healthcare courses, as well as developing and implementing courses in nutrition and business services for health professionals. Additionally, she is an accomplished writer, with many publications and conference presentations to her credit, who has served on numerous editorial review panels. Marilyn Smith-Stoner is an active member of the Editorial Board for *Home Healthcare Nurse* and the Editorial Review Committee for the *Journal of Hospice and Palliative Nursing*.

Contributors

About the Series Editor
Kay Stevens, RN, MA conceived this textbook series, and recruited and coordinated the authors in the development of each of their texts. She is the author of *Being a Health Unit Coordinator,* and the editor of a Medical-Clerical Textbook Series for Brady. Before entering education, she worked in medical/surgical and critical care nursing and in the inservice department as a clinical instructor.

Formerly a Professional Development Contract Consultant for special projects and curriculum development for the California Department of Education, Professor Stevens has also served as chairperson of the California Health Careers Statewide Advisory Committee, and been a Master Trainer for Health Careers Teacher Training through California Polytechnic University of Pomona. She also is a founding member of the National Association of Health Unit Coordinators. Professor Stevens is currently Program Coordinator of the Medical Assistant Program at Saddleback College in Mission Viejo, California, and operates her consulting business, Achiever's Development Enterprises.

Editor's Note

I would like to take this opportunity to thank the authors of this series. Their dedication and sense of mission made it a joy to work on this challenging project. I particularly wish to thank and congratulate the authors of this text, Dr. Gail Askew and Dr. Marilyn Smith-Stoner, for their professionalism and hard work on this book.

I would also like to express my sincere gratitude to the staff of Career Publishing, Inc. and most especially Valerie Harris for her professional and talented assistance throughout. I also would like to express my appreciation to Harold Haase, Publisher, for his enthusiasm for this project and for his humanistic approach to education.

Kay Stevens, RN, MA
Series Editor

Chapter One
Introduction to the Pharmacy

Objectives

After completing this chapter, you should be able to do the following:

1. Define and correctly spell each of the key terms.
2. Describe the general duties of a pharmacy clerk.
3. Identify the most important personal characteristics of a good pharmacy clerk.
4. Describe technical training that the pharmacy clerk might obtain.
5. Discuss job opportunities available to the pharmacy clerk.
6. Know the similarities and differences between inpatient pharmacies and outpatient pharmacies.
7. List some professional organizations relevant to the pharmacy.

Key Terms

- clinic
- dispense
- eligibility
- intravenous solutions (IVs)
- oral
- pharmacology
- pharmacy
- prescription
- retail pharmacy
- topical

Introduction

The last revolution of the 20th Century has been the *Biotechnical Revolution*. Biotechnology is the branch of science that uses the body's own power to produce cures or treatments for disease. As a result, the pharmacy clerk in the twenty-first century is working in one of the most exciting areas of healthcare. The field of **pharmacology** is being dramatically altered by many scientific discoveries: biologists are discovering ways of **genetically engineering** drugs for use in the treatment of many diseases; engineers are developing more and more sophisticated ways of purifying and administering drugs; and tablets, liquids, and injections are no longer the only medication routes available (Figure 1-1). The possibilities for new discoveries are endless!

pharmacology: the study of drugs and their actions.

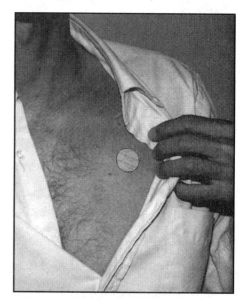

Figure 1-1: Special patches may be used to deliver medications to patients through their skin.

In addition, changes in the way healthcare is delivered are making medications more available to individuals who need them. Managed care programs such as HMO plans provide medications for little or no cost to the patient. Even Medicare patients, who normally must pay for their own medications unless the drugs are self administered (such as insulin), may choose a managed care plan instead of Medicare to pay for medication. There are many alternative methods of supplying medication. Especially important is the increasingly wide use of mail order prescription services. As a result, you may work in a **pharmacy** where you never see the patient or customer.

pharmacy: the department in a hospital, clinic, or a store in the community that dispenses medication.

Assistants in the Pharmacy and Their Titles

The principal duty of an assistant in the pharmacy is to help the pharmacist and other pharmacy staff members obtain, process, and **dispense prescriptions**, as well as other medications and supplies. However, your specific duties as an assistant in the pharmacy will depend largely on where you work. In some places, the pharmacy assistant works primarily as a clerk, and may, in fact, be called a **pharmacy clerk**. In other pharmacies, the title of aide or assistant may be used.

dispense: to provide medication as prescribed by a physician or other qualified person.

For the purposes of this text, we will be using the term, "pharmacy clerk," to describe a nonregistered, technical assistant who typically performs the following tasks:

- making and receiving telephone calls.
- handling customer service requests.
- entering computer data.
- maintaining pharmacy records.
- assisting with inventory control.
- handling customer payments.
- processing third-party billing.

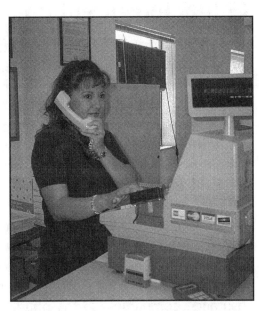

Figure 1-2: A pharmacy clerk talks to a customer on the telephone.

prescription: (often called a script) an order to dispense a medication that specifies the drug, dosage, frequency, and amount of medication to be given. It also provides information about the prescriber and the patient.

Remember that this position may be called by another term in your place of employment. Please note that a pharmacy clerk in your state may be legally restricted from performing all of these tasks—or may be able to perform more of the pharmacy technician tasks outlined in Chapter Two. Your state board of pharmacy will be able to provide you with the specific restrictions and requirements for pharmacy clerks in your state. Web site addresses for the state boards of pharmacy can be found through the National Association of Boards of Pharmacy (contact information is provided at the end of the chapter.)

retail pharmacy:
a facility that supplies prescription and nonprescription medication to customers in a particular community. It can be located in a drugstore, medical building, or grocery store, or it can be a freestanding building.

clinic:
a center, often a separate department in a hospital, that treats individuals who are patients, but have not been admitted to the hospital.

Pharmacy clerks who work in a **retail pharmacy** or **clinic** will find themselves spending the majority of their time in clerical and customer service tasks, such as sales. In a hospital pharmacy, clerks may also act as couriers, picking up medication orders and delivering medications throughout the facility. The most successful pharmacy clerks are those who take every opportunity to assist their pharmacists, technicians, and patients. Common tasks are discussed in more detail in Chapter Two.

Characteristics of Pharmacy Personnel

Individuals who work in allied healthcare, and certainly in the pharmacy, must possess specific characteristics. The most important characteristic is *trustworthiness*. Pharmacy personnel work in busy environments with a high demand for individual accountability. Medications are regulated by state and federal laws. Pharmacy personnel must be able to adhere to these regulations, as well the facility's policies. Being trustworthy with medications is one of the most significant contributions that can be made by individuals who work in healthcare, and particularly in a pharmacy.

People who work in a pharmacy also need to be *detail-oriented*. Prescriptions for medications are precise. Every part of the prescription is important. No detail is too small to check and recheck. It is also very important to be detail-oriented when verifying the source of payment for the medications. People often change insurance companies, so the pharmacy clerk needs to check the source of payment each time a customer comes into the pharmacy. Checking and rechecking addresses, telephone numbers, and other identifying information is also important to efficiency in the pharmacy.

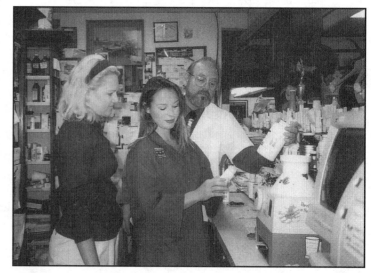

Figure 1-3: Working in a pharmacy requires teamwork.

Chapter One • Introduction to the Pharmacy

The pharmacy department is a team. All members of the team must be willing to *work together* to get the job done. Like a sports team, each member of the work team has certain jobs and limitations. The pharmacist is the head of the team. Work is carried out under his or her direction. The success of the team depends on each member doing his or her job. The pharmacy clerk plays an indispensable role on the team, by providing support to the pharmacy staff. When you have problems or questions, you should speak up about the issues. Do not wait until someone asks you. This is part of the responsibility of being on a team. This textbook and the core text of this healthcare series will help you develop the skills necessary to fulfill such responsibility.

As you might imagine, dispensing medications produces paperwork. All pharmacy personnel must have clearly *readable handwriting*. Clearly written notes and records are critical to a smooth running department. Basic computer skills are also necessary; most pharmacies are computerized. Checking prescription records, monitoring refill requests, ordering supplies, and running productivity reports are essential functions that are commonly completed using computers. When you are hired by a company, you will receive instruction on the specific computer system in use at that facility. You will need to understand how to operate the keyboard, make entries, save files, and print records. These are all standard computer skills.

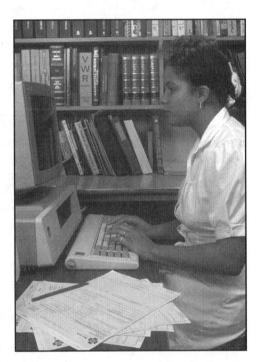

Figure 1-4: The ability to operate a computer can be a useful skill to a pharmacy clerk.

Responding to Customers with Care

All healthcare workers are in the business of helping the sick. When customers come to the pharmacy for a prescription, they place a great deal of trust in the doctor who has prescribed a certain treatment and in the pharmacy personnel who must fill that prescription. Sometimes these people may not feel well and can present a service challenge to the pharmacy clerk. People who work in the pharmacy should be patient and compassionate individuals. *Caring* means being patient when a customer is not able to recall the exact name of the medication ordered for them. When customers inquire about the progress of a prescription that they feel should have been ready right away, you are not demonstrating that you care about the customer by simply saying "come back later." Instead, take the time to find out exactly what happened and what you, and possibly the customer, must do in order to get the prescription filled as soon as possible. Often you can show compassion by simply listening to an individual without verbally responding until he or she has finished speaking.

If all of this sounds challenging, it is! Through training and practice you can acquire the skills and confidence that are necessary to be a successful pharmacy clerk.

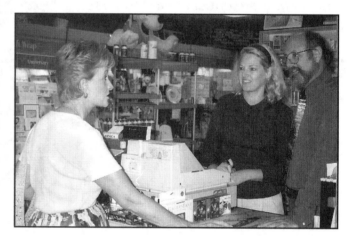

Figure 1-5: A pharmacy clerk must listen to his or her customers.

Technical Training

There are many types of training programs available for people who wish to learn the basic principles of working in the pharmacy. Some training programs for pharmacy clerks are held in traditional school environments. Others are held in vocational schools or hospitals. The cost, length of training, and educational content of the courses are individualized to the program site. Some programs are as short as four months, while others last a year.

Pharmacy clerks who want to obtain additional training in order to work as **pharmacy technicians** should look for programs based on the Model Curriculum for Pharmacy Technician Training. These programs are often accredited by the American Society of Health-System Pharmacists (ASHP). ASHP-accredited programs meet national standards for quality in pharmacy technician training.

Like pharmacy clerk training, pharmacy technician training programs are varied, with some certificate programs as brief as six months. Other schools offer two-year programs, which allow students to earn their degrees as pharmacy technicians. Pharmacy technician training places more emphasis on the technical skills required in the hospital pharmacy. Technician training programs include both lecture and lab activities designed to develop these necessary technical skills. Many programs also require the technician trainee to complete an "experiential" training component, called an internship or an externship, in an actual pharmacy.

In some states, there is a career ladder between the pharmacy clerk and pharmacy technician position. For example, current law in California allows a pharmacy clerk with 1500 hours of pharmacy clerk experience to apply for registration as a pharmacy technician. In this case, it is the pharmacist's responsibility to train the pharmacy clerk to work as a technician. Technicians who are trained in this manner work primarily in retail pharmacies, since they have not learned the specialized skills needed for hospital employment.

Wherever the clerk begins his or her training, a foundation for later learning is formed. The clerk's duty to provide good customer service must be the center of each learning experience and every task performed while assisting the pharmacy team. The pharmacist and pharmacy technician also focus on customer service, but have considerably expanded roles based on their level of education. A firm foundation in customer service and retail operations will give you important skills for more advanced jobs in the pharmacy.

Places of Employment

Finding a job as a pharmacy clerk involves researching your local community medical facilities (Figure 1-6). The two main practice environments for pharmacy clerks are **outpatient pharmacies** (in independent retail drug stores, clinics, or large retail chains) and **inpatient pharmacies** (in hospitals). However, many areas now have specialized pharmacies that do not serve the general public. Often called "closed-door" pharmacies, these include mail-order pharmacies and centralized refill pharmacies. Other specialized pharmacies service home health agencies that provide intravenous fluids and medications for administration to patients in their homes. Still others serve patients in long-term care and rehabilitation centers. All of these facilities are potential places of employment.

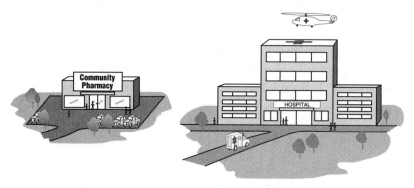

Figure 1-6: There are two main types of pharmacies: inpatient pharmacies and outpatient pharmacies.

Individuals with certain physical challenges may find working in a pharmacy to be a suitable career. For example, the work environment in a pharmacy might be modified to accommodate a wheelchair or other mobility device. Many county and state agencies provide funding for workplace designs that allow the physically challenged to work effectively; contact these resources for further information. The Job Accommodation Network, or JAN, can also provide information on pharmacies that employ people with physical challenges.

Their address is:

JAN, WVU
809 Allen Hall
PO Box 6122
Morgantown, WI 26506-6122

The Hospital Environment

Hospital pharmacies are very different from retail drug stores, or community pharmacies. In the hospital, the customers are patients and their **eligibility** for insurance has been verified by the admitting or billing offices. The pharmacy staff rarely needs to follow-up on a bill. Once the charge is processed in the hospital billing system, another department follows through with collection of money owed.

The medication needs of patients change very rapidly in the hospital. Medication deliveries to patients' units or nursing stations will take up a large part of the pharmacy clerk's job duties. Exchanging and stocking medications that are kept on reserve in the nursing units are also very important aspects of the job. **Intravenous solutions (IVs)** are used extensively in the hospital. The pharmacy clerk will become familiar with many types of administration systems for IVs.

Physicians are in much closer contact with the pharmacy staff in a hospital than in a retail pharmacy. They will often call the pharmacist to get advice on medications. When multiple physicians are consulting for one patient, the pharmacist will frequently serve as the *clearing house* for the various medications ordered for the patient. This minimizes the chances for mistakes in the patient's medication schedule.

eligibility: satisfaction of all of an insurance company's requirements to become qualified to receive insurance benefits.

intravenous solutions (IVs): sterile fluids that are injected directly into a vein. These solutions may contain medications, nutrients, or supplements that aid in the body's normal functioning.

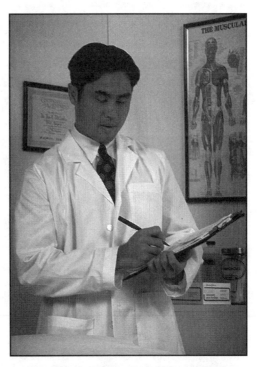

Figure 1-7: Physicians depend on the hospital pharmacy to help coordinate medications for patients who have more than one doctor.

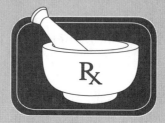

The Concerns of Key People Who Affect the Hospital Pharmacy

TITLE	CONCERN
Hospital Administrator	Is the department making money? Are state, local, and federal regulations being met? Are patients being served?
Controller/Risk Manager	Are necessary supplies available? Are all charges accurate? Are prescriptions filled accurately? Are policies followed?
Nursing Service	Is the correct medication being administered? Is the medication available on time? Is the medication easily given to patients?
Medical Staff	Is the medication being given to the patient as ordered? Is the medication available? Is the medication effective?
Patients/Customers	Is the medication effective? Does the medication produce unwanted side effects? Is the medication affordable?
Insurance Carrier	Is the medication effective? Is the medication too expensive?

Figure 1-8: The Concerns of Key People Who Affect the Hospital Pharmacy

The Outpatient Pharmacy

Outpatient pharmacies are often as busy as their hospital counterparts. However, there is a difference in the type, frequency, and urgency of the medication needs of the customers. In addition, the billing and collecting of fees for medications makes up a much larger part of the job.

Medications dispensed through the outpatient pharmacy tend to concentrate on **oral** and **topical** medications. While frequently used in home care, IV solutions (which constitute a large part of a hospital pharmacy's business) tend to be centralized in specialized home infusion pharmacies. Large pharmacies benefit from robotic machines that count and dispense tablets, capsules, and so on. This speeds up the process of filling prescription bottles and increases accuracy at the same time.

oral: refers to the mouth. In the pharmacy, it refers to medication given by mouth.

topical: refers to the surface of the body. In the pharmacy, it refers to the application of medications to the surface of the body.

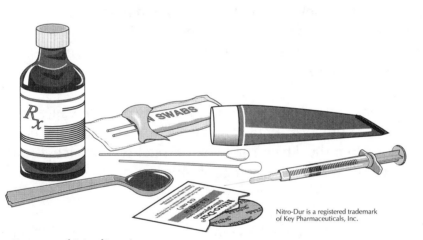

Figure 1-9: Forms of Medication

Whereas the hospital pharmacist often provides advice to physicians, the outpatient pharmacist is more likely to provide advice to customers. Dispensing prescriptions, verifying unclear orders, and participating in the direct business management of the pharmacy will be a much larger part of the job for this pharmacist.

Other Types of Pharmacies

Mail-order pharmacies are becoming an increasingly large part of the pharmacy industry. Often they are part of managed care organizations or advocacy groups. The American Association for Retired Persons maintains one of the largest mail-order pharmacies in the country. Such pharmacies succeed because they deliver high volumes of medication to many people. Often the medications are those taken for chronic conditions, such as heart and lung diseases, diabetes, and other long-term conditions.

Central refill pharmacies are also becoming common in some areas of the country. This type of pharmacy uses automation to fill large numbers of prescription refills for distribution to chain drug stores or HMO clinics. Patients may not realize that their refill was actually processed at a central refill pharmacy, since they pick up the medication at their local chain drug store. Pharmacy personnel who work in a central refill location will seldom interact directly with the customers or patients. Most refill orders are transmitted through voice mail or on-line computer refill systems.

Specialty pharmacies meet very specific needs, often serving a large geographical area. The primary example of a specialty pharmacy is the *home healthcare pharmacy*. Home healthcare provides hospital-type services to patients in their homes. Hospice care and home infusion are examples of home healthcare services.

Much of the business of a home healthcare pharmacy will involve providing intravenous medications for patients. Infusion fluids, antibiotic doses, pain management, and nutritional support make up the majority of these medication orders. Home care patients frequently have special catheters inserted into their veins to allow delivery of IV products over long periods of time.

Another type of specialty pharmacy deals with *chemotherapy* drugs. Used for cancer treatment, chemotherapy drugs require very specialized handling due to their toxicity. As a result, some communities have pharmacies that deal exclusively with chemotherapy medications for delivery to hospitals, clinics, and home healthcare agencies.

Specialty pharmacies receive most of their orders directly from the prescriber or through a home healthcare agency. There is little face-to-face contact with patients in these pharmacies.

Professional Organizations

There are many national professional organizations that can provide you with information about pharmacy. These organizations distribute information on new drugs, new laws, and new methods of providing pharmaceutical care to patients. These organizations also set standards of practice, which often serve as the basis for the policies you'll follow at work. The two largest organizations that represent the interests of pharmacists are the American Pharmaceutical Association (APhA) and the American Society of Health-System Pharmacists (ASHP). Both of these national groups have state and local affiliated chapters.

Pharmacy technicians also have national organizations representing their interests. The first of these organizations is the American Association of Pharmacy Technicians (AAPT). AAPT has affiliated chapters in many areas. More recently, the National Pharmacy Technicians Association (NPTA) was formed.

Pharmacy educators are also represented by a national group: the American Association of Colleges of Pharmacy (AACP). If you are ultimately interested in training to be a pharmacist, AACP can provide you with essential information.

Pharmacy practice is regulated by both state and federal law and by the rules and regulations enacted by the state Boards of Pharmacy. The various professional organizations employ lobbyists who present and promote pharmacy-related legislation at the state and federal levels. The federal government agencies that regulate medications are outlined in Chapter Four.

Web Sites

American Association of Colleges of Pharmacy	*www.aacp.org*
American Association of Pharmacy Technicians	*www.pharmacytechnician.com*
American Pharmaceutical Association	*www.aphanet.org*
American Society of Health-System Pharmacists	*www.ashp.org*
National Association of Boards of Pharmacy	*www.nabp.net*
National Pharmacy Technicians Association	*www.pharmacytechnician.org*
Pharmacy Technician Certification Board	*www.ptcb.org*
Pharmacy Technician Educators Council	*www.rxptec.org*

Chapter Summary

The healthcare industry is constantly changing, as technology and financial constraints modify the way services are provided. Our aging population and the development of new drugs present pharmacies with the additional challenge of dealing with large increases in prescription demand.

To fill the growing number of prescriptions, pharmacies have made a number of changes in the way they operate. Some of the changes include hiring more ancillary personnel, such as pharmacy clerks and technicians; centralizing pharmacy services; and using automation and robotic systems.

In addition to the traditional drug store or hospital pharmacy, you may find yourself working in a mail-order, central fill, or other type of specialized pharmacy. Regardless of where you work, you will be interacting with pharmacists and pharmacy technicians to provide pharmaceutical care. To be a successful pharmacy clerk, you will need to have certain characteristics. You will need to be trustworthy, detail-oriented, and able to work well with others. You must also have readable handwriting. In addition, it is important to be patient and compassionate, so that others recognize that you are a caring individual.

This is a challenging time to be working in the healthcare industry. Your future as a pharmacy clerk promises to be interesting and exciting!

Chapter One • Introduction to the Pharmacy   1-15

Name _____
Date _____

Student Enrichment Activities

Complete the following exercises.

1. List four personal characteristics necessary for success in the pharmacy field.
   A. _____   C. _____
   B. _____   D. _____

2. Add four personal characteristics you possess that would be beneficial in the pharmacy.
   A. _____   C. _____
   B. _____   D. _____

3. Describe three duties of the pharmacy clerk.
   A. _____
   B. _____
   C. _____

4. What are the two main environments in which a pharmacy clerk can work?
   A. _____   B. _____

Define the following words.

5. pharmacology: _____
   _____

6. prescription: _____
   _____
   _____

7. dispense: _____
   _____

Name three professional organizations associated with the pharmacy.

8. _____

9. _____

10. _____

Match each description in Column A with the appropriate letter in Column B. List all letters that apply. Some letters may be used more than once.

Column A

11. ____ Pharmacy clerk duties

12. ____ Pharmacies that employ pharmacy clerks

13. ____ A type of pharmacy found in a hospital

14. ____ The study of drugs and their effects

15. ____ The head of the pharmacy team

16. ____ The most important trait in a pharmacy clerk

17. ____ A type of pharmacy found in supermarkets or clinics

18. ____ A position that requires more education than a pharmacy clerk, and less education than a pharmacist

Column B

A. pharmacology

B. stocking shelves

C. pharmacist

D. paperwork

E. good handwriting

F. inpatient pharmacy

G. outpatient pharmacy

H. pharmacy technician

I. trustworthiness

J. customer service

K. assist the pharmacist

Chapter Two
The Pharmacy Team

Objectives

After completing this chapter, you should be able to do the following:

1. Define and correctly spell each of the key terms.
2. List the members of the pharmacy team.
3. Explain the roles of each team member in the pharmacy.
4. Explain the basic pharmacy organizational plan.

Key Terms

- accounting
- accounts payable
- accounts receivable
- certification
- compliance
- CPhT
- over-the-counter (OTC)
- pharmaceutical care
- pharmacist
- pharmacy clerk
- pharmacy technician

Introduction

Pharmacies are located in a variety of facilities and communities. However, the basic organizational structure of each is similar. This chapter will introduce you to the most commonly employed personnel in a pharmacy. Variations in this description will be based on the size, customer type, and community needs for the pharmacy itself.

There is no one *right* way to run a pharmacy. There is also no minimum or maximum number of employees working for a pharmacy. Considerable variation in practice is likely to be found in every community and setting. The way in which a pharmacy is organized depends largely upon the type of customers served by the pharmacy. Common to all pharmacies, however, is the need for the employees to work together as a team to provide good **pharmaceutical care** to the customers or patients.

pharmaceutical care: services that improve a patient's health through the appropriate use of medications.

pharmacist: someone who is trained and licensed to evaluate medication use, prepare and dispense medications, and provide counseling and drug information to patients and healthcare workers.

The Pharmacist

Pharmacists receive their professional education at pharmacy schools located in major universities throughout the United States. Although many practicing pharmacists earned Bachelor of Science (BS) degrees in pharmacy, most current pharmacy students will earn the Doctor of Pharmacy (or **PharmD**) degree. The PharmD is a professional doctorate; pharmacists who have earned the PharmD degree may use the title "Dr." before their names.

Most PharmD programs require the completion of at least two years of prerequisite college courses, followed by four years in the school of pharmacy. Accelerated and nontraditional PharmD programs are also available at some schools. All states require that pharmacist candidates complete an internship, in addition to their college degree.

Pharmacists must pass a rigorous licensing exam before they can begin to practice their profession. Many states rely on the national licensing exam, the NAPLEX, although some states have developed their own board exams. Once licensed, pharmacists may use the initials **RPh** after their names, to indicate that they are "registered pharmacists."

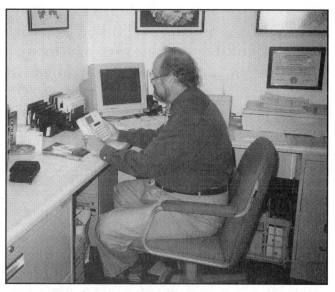

Figure 2-1: The pharmacist has many duties in addition to dispensing medications, such as monitoring cholesterol and blood sugar levels for customers.

The focus of pharmacist education has shifted as the role of the pharmacist has changed. At the turn of the 20th century, pharmacists spent their days extracting chemicals and compounding medicines from raw ingredients. Pharmacist education in those days consisted of courses in pharmacognosy (recognizing and using plants as drugs) and in learning to prepare different types of dosage forms. Pharmacists learned to make ointments and suppositories, to roll out "pills," and to punch capsules. The pharmacists then dispensed these products to fill prescriptions.

When the drug manufacturing companies took over the preparation of most drugs, the pharmacist's dispensing function was reduced to "counting and pouring" pre-made medications. By the turn of the 21st century, pharmacy technicians were doing the "counting and pouring" in many states.

So what do pharmacists do now? Pharmacists are the drug information experts of the healthcare system. Pharmacists work with **prescribers** (physicians, osteopaths, dentists, physician's assistants, and nurse practitioners) to help select the best medications for their patients. While hospital and clinic pharmacists are able to do this in person, many pharmacists do their consulting work by phone or through computer links with prescribers in their offices.

Pharmacists interpret and evaluate prescription orders for accuracy, completeness, and availability. Pharmacists monitor each prescription for appropriateness by performing a **drug utilization review (DUR)**, which involves checking for drug allergies and for interactions between medications. Some pharmacists also monitor how well a medication works for a patient. For example, a pharmacist may monitor a patient's response to a blood pressure medication by checking the patient's blood pressure. Under certain protocols, a pharmacist may even make adjustments to the drug therapy based on the patient's response.

In addition to acting as an information resource for medical personnel, pharmacists provide counseling directly to patients. By providing patient education on prescription and **over-the-counter (OTC)** medications, pharmacists can help assure **compliance**. With the increase in use of alternative medicine, many pharmacists also counsel patients on the use of vitamins and herbal remedies.

Of course, pharmacists still fill prescriptions, especially in states that do not yet permit pharmacy technicians to do so. Pharmacists still compound specialized medications that are not made by the drug manufacturing companies. And pharmacists are responsible for instructing and directing other personnel in the completion of their pharmacy-related duties. In states that allow pharmacy technicians to dispense, pharmacists are legally responsible for the accuracy of the technician's work.

Pharmacy schools now prepare pharmacy students for these expanded roles with increased emphasis on life sciences, pharmacology, and communications skills. However, pharmacists are never done with their training. As new drugs and new therapies are developed by the pharmaceutical industry, pharmacists must keep up. Most pharmacists subscribe to professional journals and attend continuing education seminars to keep themselves informed of new developments. Often these journals and seminar programs are left in the pharmacy for interested employees to read.

over-the-counter (OTC): refers to nonprescription medications that can be purchased in most drugstores and some supermarkets.

compliance: taking a medication accurately, according to its directions for use.

Chapter Two • The Pharmacy Team

2-5

The pharmacist is one of the most trusted professionals in the community. The public is well aware of the need for competence in handling prescription medications. Pharmacists are equally aware of the public trust given to them. As a pharmacy clerk, you can help guarantee that your pharmacist and pharmacy are seen in a positive light. Providing good customer relations, as well as proper prescription services, will result in a continued positive image of the pharmacy profession.

The Pharmacy Technician

Pharmacy technicians work at an intermediate level on the pharmacy team. Technicians usually have more training and responsibility than pharmacy clerks. However, technicians do not have the professional education or legal responsibilities of the pharmacist. While pharmacy technicians are highly trained in the technical aspects of handling medications, they do not perform tasks that require professional judgment. Pharmacy technicians work primarily with the drug product, whereas pharmacists concentrate more on the drug information aspects of pharmaceutical care.

pharmacy technician: an allied health worker with advanced on-the-job training and/or education, who assists the pharmacist and customers (training and education requirements vary among the states).

Typical pharmacy technician tasks are regulated by state law and vary by practice site, but may include:

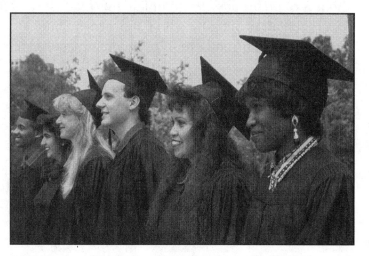

Figure 2-2: Pharmacy technicians may obtain an Associate's degree from a community college.

- selecting, counting, and pouring prescription medications.
- updating patient profiles and preparing prescription labels.
- assisting with drug purchasing and inventory control.
- packaging medications in unit-dose or med-card form.
- mixing intravenous solutions and other specialized medications.
- gathering data for pharmacists to use in monitoring drug therapy.

Pharmacy technicians also assist with clerical duties, such as filing pharmacy records, answering the telephone, directing calls, and operating the cash register. In some retail pharmacies, a pharmacy technician acts as the business manager, handling insurance billing, staff scheduling, and a variety of other business-related tasks.

Although pharmacy technician training requirements vary from state to state, the trend is toward requiring the completion of some type of formal training program. As discussed in Chapter One, pharmacy technician training can be obtained at a variety of educational sites, from high school career programs to community colleges offering an associate degree. A comprehensive list of technician training programs is available through the Pharmacy Technician Educators Council (PTEC). The American Society of Health-System Pharmacists maintains a list of ASHP-accredited training programs on its web site.

Pharmacy technicians are registered or licensed to practice by some state boards of pharmacy. To complete this process, a technician applicant submits documentation of training and undergoes a background check. However, most states do not currently require pharmacy technicians to pass a state licensing exam.

certification: demonstration of knowledge and abilities.

CPhT: certified pharmacy technician; one who has passed the national PTCB exam.

In order to assess the competency of pharmacy technicians, the Pharmacy Technician Certification Board (PTCB) has developed a national **certification** test. Technicians who pass the PTCB exam are considered to be "certified" pharmacy technicians and are entitled to use the initials **CPhT** after their names. While certification is voluntary in most states, the movement to require certification is growing. In any case, becoming a CPhT should be the goal of all pharmacy technicians.

The pressure to contain healthcare costs has led to many new career opportunities for pharmacy technicians. By using technicians to handle the product-related pharmacy tasks, pharmacists are free to spend more time in drug information and patient care activities. Well-qualified pharmacy technicians are essential to the modern practice of pharmacy.

The Pharmacy Clerk

Pharmacy clerks complement the work of the pharmacist and the pharmacy technician in a variety of ways. As discussed in Chapter One, the work of the pharmacy clerk often consists of extensive clerical and customer service activities. Typical pharmacy clerk tasks include the following:

- waiting on customers.
- receiving prescriptions.
- answering the telephone.
- entering computer data.
- preparing prescription labels.
- filing pharmacy records.
- stocking shelves.
- filling orders for non-prescription (OTC) drugs and supplies.
- handling customer payments.
- verifying insurance coverage.
- processing third-party billings.
- transporting medications in hospitals.

pharmacy clerk: an allied health worker who works in a pharmacy assisting the pharmacist and customers.

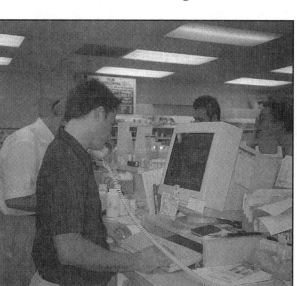

Figure 2-3: Well-trained pharmacy clerks provide valuable services to pharmacists, such as checking for prescription refills on the computer.

Remember that state law may restrict the tasks that a pharmacy clerk may perform in your state. This is particularly true as it relates to the preparation of prescription labels and the handling of medications.

Pharmacy clerks, like pharmacy technicians, benefit from the challenge to contain costs in healthcare. Well-trained clerks provide valuable services for the pharmacy team. This, in turn, increases the efficiency of the whole pharmacy.

Pharmacy clerks also have much of the responsibility for customer satisfaction. The pharmacy clerk is usually the first person the customers see. The customers' first impression of the pharmacy will depend on the image the pharmacy clerk projects. Keeping the customers satisfied means they will return to the same pharmacy over and over again for their medication needs. Such repeat business is the foundation for a successful retail pharmacy.

The Prescriber

A description of the pharmacy team would not be complete without including the physicians and other healthcare professionals who prescribe medications. Prescribers are the driving force behind all pharmacies, because they originate the orders for medication. As a result, pharmacy personnel should consider prescribers as members of the team, even though they are not usually present in the pharmacy.

Prescribers rely on the skills of all pharmacy personnel to help them with prescription orders. A mutually respectful relationship ensures that patients and customers will get the medications they need in a timely manner. The prescriber initiates this process by prescribing a medication. The pharmacy staff completes the process by preparing the medication for use by the patient.

Most prescriptions are written by physicians, although certain other professionals are legally qualified to prescribe medications. Dentists, podiatrists, veterinarians, and optometrists may be able to prescribe medications that fall within their "scope of practice." For example, dentists often prescribe antibiotics for tooth and gum infections or analgesics for dental pain. Veterinarians can only prescribe medications for use by animals, although these prescriptions may be sent to the pharmacy to be filled.

Physician's assistants and nurse practitioners, who work under the supervision of physicians in clinics and group practices, also have prescribing rights under certain circumstances. In some states, pharmacists can also prescribe under specific protocols. This expansion of the definition of "prescriber" is designed to make healthcare more available to patients.

Pharmacies are receiving prescription orders in different ways now, as well as from different types of prescribers. The written prescription, delivered to the pharmacy by the patient, is still the most common, followed by telephone prescription orders. However, prescriptions are now received by FAX and by direct computer link as well. Regardless of how the prescription order arrives, the patient still relies on the pharmacy team to provide the medication accurately and quickly.

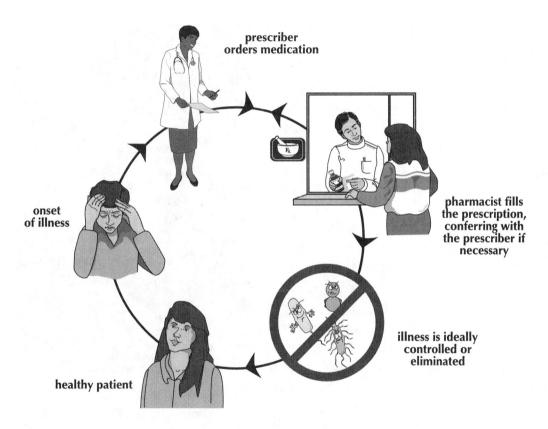

Figure 2-4: How Medications are Prescribed and Filled

The Business Manager

One of the many healthcare revolutions in progress focuses on the process of integrating standard business practices into the healthcare industry. Workers in the medical field have not been used to thinking of themselves as being involved in a business. However, healthcare is the BUSINESS OF TAKING CARE OF PEOPLE.

accounting: a system of record keeping that tracks business transactions, such as money owed by customers and money spent for operating costs.

Business managers are becoming increasingly important to pharmacies. They are already an indispensable part of many large pharmacies. The business manager is primarily concerned with customer service, **accounting**, personnel practices, and insurance reimbursement. Business managers acquire and maintain contracts with managed health organizations that provide large amounts of business. With the huge growth of health maintenance organizations (HMOs), the volume of business provided by HMOs and other types of managed care plans is often essential to the financial success of a pharmacy. Some business managers may also be involved in acquiring contracts with specialty pharmacies that focus on intravenous fluids and medication, chemotherapy for cancer treatment, or with long term care facilities. Contracting is a complicated and essential function for any financially sound pharmacy.

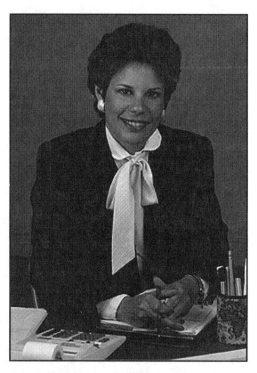

Figure 2-5: The business manager is becoming increasingly important to pharmacies.

accounts receivable: money owed by a customer or other debtor on a current debt.

The financial component of the business manager's job may involve most of his or her time. **Accounts receivable** are payments owed to the pharmacy. These come mainly from prepaid health plans such as HMOs. These plans provide a prescription benefit to their plan members. When one of these customers uses the services of the pharmacy, the bill is paid by their prepaid plan or insurance company. Thus, the business manager keeps track of these sales and collects money from the proper plan or company.

Accounts payable are accounts on which the pharmacy owes money. These include utility bills, supply bills, and bills for the medications themselves which are supplied by drug companies. The business manager makes sure that bills are paid on time and correctly. Often it is the business manager who processes time cards and ensures that the staff members are paid appropriately for their work.

accounts payable: money owed by a business to creditors such as suppliers or other businesses.

Drug Suppliers and Salespeople

Sales representatives for drug companies are a familiar sight in pharmacies. They are employed by drug manufacturers to promote their products. The sales representative's job is to influence the medication-related recommendations pharmacists and physicians make to patients.

Representatives of drug suppliers provide valuable services to healthcare providers. These services include bringing information on new drugs and methods of administering drugs. They also provide samples of medications and a wide variety of patient education material. Orders for medication may also be placed through these salespeople.

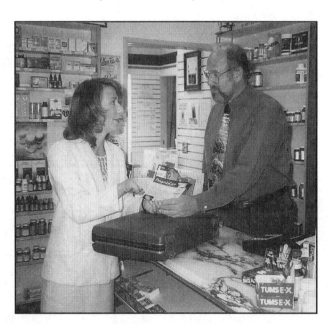

Figure 2-6: Pharmaceutical salespeople can be valuable sources of information to pharmacists.

Other Healthcare Workers

Many other healthcare workers interact with the pharmacy staff. Nurses, therapists, and office workers are often in contact with pharmacy personnel. Successful pharmacy personnel recognize the valuable and unique contributions of all the people with whom they work. Making it a policy to consider all other healthcare workers as part of the team is an important part of maintaining smooth working relationships.

The Organizational Structure of a Pharmacy

An organizational chart that shows the relationship among key members of a typical hospital, or inpatient, pharmacy team is described in Figure 2-7. A similar chart for outpatient pharmacies is shown in Figure 2-8. This will vary depending on the job description for each employee. Many employers will provide a department organizational chart and job description for a job applicant. This material can be valuable to you in discussing the job with potential employers. When interviewing for a job, be sure to ask for a job description and the organizational plan of the pharmacy.

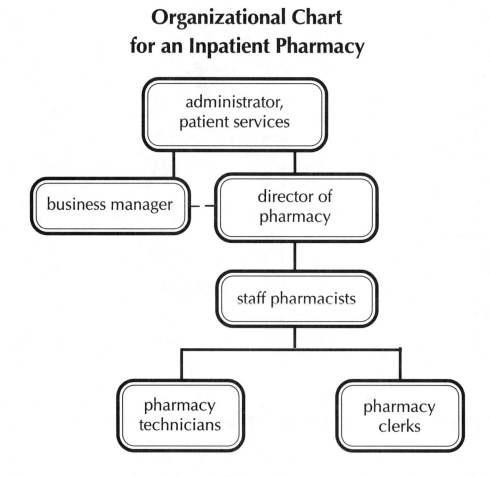

Figure 2-7: The Organizational Structure of an Inpatient Pharmacy

Chapter Two • The Pharmacy Team 2-13

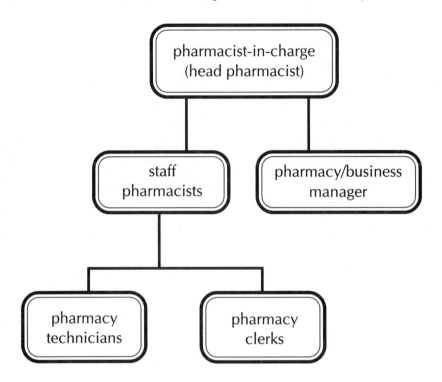

Figure 2-8: The Organizational Structure of an Outpatient Pharmacy

Chapter Summary

Working in a pharmacy, whether it is in the hospital or community, means teamwork. The pharmacist, the technician, and the clerk form the core of the pharmacy team. Prescribers, nurses, and other healthcare workers can be part of the extended pharmacy team. The pharmacy team shares a common goal: *To provide good pharmaceutical care to the patients.*

Each member of the pharmacy team has certain specific tasks to perform, but each shares some duties with other team members. Each team member must be able to count on the others to do their jobs. Being aware of each team member's unique role in relation to your own will assist you in performing your job in an efficient and rewarding manner. As a pharmacy clerk, you have an important contribution to make to the pharmacy team.

Chapter Two • The Pharmacy Team 2-15

Name _____
Date _____

Student Enrichment Activities

Fill in the blanks.

1. Pharmacists must pass a rigorous _____ _____, such as the _____, before practicing their profession.

2. Healthcare is the _____ of taking care of people.

3. Physicians, dentists, veterinarians, and optometrists are all examples of a _____.

4. The organizational structure of an inpatient pharmacy includes the _____, the _____ _____, the _____, the _____ _____, the pharmacy _____, and _____.

5. _____ _____ provide samples of medications and patient educational materials.

6. _____ is a system of financial record keeping.

Match the terms in Column A with the appropriate description in Column B.

Column A

7. _____ RPh

8. _____ OTC

9. _____ physician's assistant

10. _____ business manager

11. _____ accounts receivable

12. _____ CPhT

13. _____ accounts payable

14. _____ compliance

15. _____ PharmD

Column B

A. designation for a certified pharmacy technician

B. the amount of money owed to a pharmacy

C. the amount of money the pharmacy owes to suppliers

D. over-the-counter medications

E. taking a medication accurately, according to its directions for use

F. concerned with the customer service and accounting aspects of a pharmacy

G. indicates a registered pharmacist

H. can write prescriptions under certain circumstances

I. a degree in pharmacy

Chapter Three
Essential Skills and Responsibilities

Objectives

After completing this chapter, you should be able to do the following:

1. Define and correctly spell each of the key terms.

2. List the steps of effective communication.

3. Explain the principles of basic hygiene and safety in the pharmacy.

4. Describe the operation of the cash register and credit card scanner in the pharmacy.

5. Describe a properly filled out check.

6. Understand insurance terms that are used in the pharmacy.

Key Terms

- controlled substance
- copayment
- coverage
- cross-contamination
- customer service
- formulary
- hygiene
- ineligible
- insured
- narcotic
- outpatient
- sharps container
- STAT
- third-party payor

Introduction

This chapter will describe the importance of good customer service, effective communication, and other duties of the pharmacy clerk. Being a successful pharmacy clerk means mastering a variety of skills. Some skills are technical skills, but most skills pertain to customer service, organization, and staff relations.

Customer Service

customer service: courteous assistance provided to a customer as determined by his or her needs.

Customer service begins with the first words spoken to the patient, physician, or healthcare worker who enters or calls the pharmacy. In most pharmacies, calls are first received by the pharmacy clerk. If you are answering the telephone, be sure that you are ready to take information. Paper and pencils or pens should always be available to take notes. If it is within your job description to check on a prescription refill, be sure to be near a computer terminal to answer questions promptly and accurately.

When answering a telephone, it is important to identify yourself, provide the name of your pharmacy or department, and greet the customer. In a retail pharmacy, an appropriate greeting might be, *"Main Street Pharmacy. This is Marilyn. How can I help you?"* Your tone of voice will tell the caller a great deal about your interest in helping him or her. Speak clearly and in a pleasant tone.

Chapter Three • Essential Skills and Responsibilities

If a caller does not identify himself or herself, be sure to ask for a name. This is especially important before you put the caller on hold. When starting a new job, ask for an orientation session on how to use the telephone system. Make sure you understand how to put callers on hold, how to transfer calls, and any other special considerations in answering the phone.

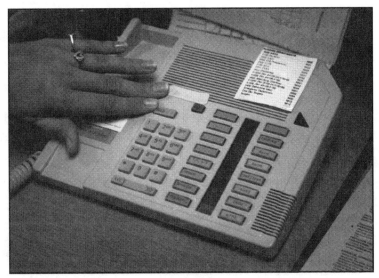

Figure 3-1: The phone system in most pharmacies will have multiple phone lines.

If the customer is calling for information, be clear in your own mind as to what kind of information is needed. For instance, does the person need to speak to a pharmacist for a medication question, or does he or she need to contact the business manager in order to get information about a bill? You will only be able to properly direct the customer if you have taken the time to get the pertinent information. The following is the information you will need from a customer who requires additional help:

1. The caller's name and the patient's name, if different. Be sure to get the correct spellings.

2. A phone number, or numbers, where the caller can be reached. Ask how long the caller will be at each number, in case a return call is necessary much later in the day.

3. The reason for the call.

    a. Is the call from a doctor's office? Calls from doctor's offices have priority and many require the immediate attention of the pharmacist.

    b. Is this an urgent request, or can it be handled as time allows?

c. Is this a prescription refill? Obtain the prescription number and, if possible, the name of the medication. If the refill is for someone other than the caller (for example, a family member), be sure to ask for the patient's name.

d. Is the caller requesting medication that has not yet been prescribed? Obtain the doctor's name and telephone number. If the caller has spoken to a specific person in the doctor's office, ask for that person's name also.

e. Does the caller have a billing question? Get the customer's pharmacy account number or the insurance company name and identification number.

f. Does the caller want to place a special order for over-the-counter medications or supplies? Be sure to ask for the complete product name and the size or quantity desired.

Customer service is also important in a clinic or hospital pharmacy. While other clinic or hospital departments may not purchase pharmacy services directly, the pharmacy clerk should still consider them to be customers. Quality patient care depends on good services from all related departments. Therefore, every department employee should perform functions as if he or she were marketing services to customers, no matter who is paying for the service.

In a hospital or clinic pharmacy it is usually enough to answer the phone with the department name and your name. For example, an appropriate greeting might be, *"Pharmacy. Marilyn speaking."* To help clarify communications, you may be asked to use your position title along with your name. In this case, the greeting would be, *"Pharmacy. This is pharmacy clerk Marilyn."*

STAT: Now! This order or request must be handled immediately.

Since hospital departments often are dealing with emergency situations, the urgency of the call is very important to assess. If the caller's request is **STAT**, it must be handled immediately. STAT requests are often defined as those that must be carried out within 15 to 20 minutes, or sooner. They should be given your first priority. Requests that are "ASAP" must be taken care of "as soon as possible," with a maximum of one hour in many facilities.

Chapter Three • Essential Skills and Responsibilities

The same basic information should be obtained from callers to a clinic or hospital pharmacy as is outlined above. In addition, the pharmacy clerk should also obtain:

1. The location of the caller and the patient. (For example: the department, ward, or room number.)

2. The patient's medical record or case number.

If it is necessary to put the customer on hold, be sure to ask the customer if you may put him or her on hold first and, on obtaining his or her permission, press the hold button down firmly. This action will avoid hanging up on the customer. If there are multiple lines on the telephone you are using, be sure to make a note of who is holding on each of the lines. On a busy morning in the pharmacy, it is easy to lose track of things like this. Ensuring that callers do not have to identify themselves several times is an important part of good customer service.

If a customer is on hold for a certain length of time, most telephones will begin to ring again. This interval is usually between 45 seconds and one minute. If this happens, ask the caller if he or she wishes to continue to hold. Most experts say a caller should not be on hold for more than one minute without an update. Time is very valuable to everyone. Make sure customers know you are concerned enough about them to limit their time on hold.

If you are taking a message, give the caller the following information:

- Your name.
- The name of the person who will be contacting the caller and some indication of when a return call or access to the appropriate person can be expected. (Be sure to ask where the caller will be at that time and obtain that telephone or pager number.)
- The length of time he or she should wait before contacting the pharmacy for assistance if no response is received.
- The closing time of the pharmacy (if it is close to that time).

If a customer becomes upset or is difficult to deal with, remember that some people come to a pharmacy feeling sick. If someone is picking up the medication for the patient, he or she is often close to and concerned about the patient. Delays in obtaining the necessary medication mean that a patient may experience prolonged pain or other discomforts. This additional time, although it may only be a few minutes, adds to the stress of an illness. Being sensitive to the stressful situation caused by a person being sick will ensure that you do as much as you can to get a prescription filled as quickly and efficiently as possible.

In Real Life...

Maria began working as a pharmacy clerk for the Community Hospital pharmacy 3 months ago. She has become familiar with all the departments of the hospital and knows who to contact when questions come up that are beyond her job description.

Recently, the hospital opened a new **outpatient** pharmacy window and there have been delays in filling the outpatient prescriptions. These delays have usually been during periods when there are emergencies in the intensive care units and on days when certain surgeries are performed.

Tuesdays and Thursdays have been the two days of the week when most of the delays have occurred. Special surgeries are scheduled for those days. These surgeries strain the ability to provide services in other areas of the pharmacy. If an emergency occurs elsewhere in the hospital, it is certain to cause a backup in the pharmacy.

On Thursday the pharmacy is busy as usual. Maria gets a call that two patients in the Intensive Care Unit have had additional complications, and new pharmacy orders are on the way. Maria realizes that the pharmacy will be providing many additional medications, including time-consuming intravenous medications, to the intensive care units. The outpatient window is scheduled to open in 15 minutes. Maria can see that four people are already lined up to have their prescriptions filled.

outpatient: a patient who receives treatment from a healthcare facility without being admitted to a hospital.

Discussion Questions

1. What can Maria do to prepare for the first customers?

2. Are there some things that Maria can do to prepare for possible delays in getting prescriptions filled?

3. Should Maria tell the customers outright that their prescriptions will be delayed?

4. Is it good customer relations to tell the people to come back later?

Chapter Three • Essential Skills and Responsibilities

In the preceding example, the pharmacy clerk can begin to develop a plan to service the outpatient customers by bringing the situation to the attention of the head pharmacist.

In Real Life...

> Maria tells Alex, the supervisor for the day, that there has been a pattern of long delays in filling outpatient prescriptions on Thursdays. Maria also explains what she feels is the cause. Since there are only 15 minutes until the outpatient pharmacy opens, Maria has to be brief. Using the time to complain about the customer load would cause even more delays in providing good customer service, since there would be no time left to arrive at a solution to the problem.
>
> Alex tells Maria that he hadn't realized the delays were becoming routine. He promises to look into ways of preventing this in the future. In order to minimize delays this time, Alex instructs Maria to get additional information on all the customers today. He tells her to ask each customer how long they are able to wait for a prescription, if necessary. Based on this information, Maria is to give the most urgent prescriptions to the pharmacy staff first. Next, Maria is to ask customers if they have any additional business in the hospital. If they are also going to another department, she suggests they attend to that business while waiting. She also promises to call that department and let them know when the prescription is ready. Before the customer leaves, she asks if he or she needs directions to that department, and provides information when needed. If the customer has no other errands in the hospital, Maria suggests the person get some refreshments in the cafeteria. Once again, she makes arrangements to call them in the cafeteria to let them know when the prescription is ready.
>
> Maria has made it clear to the customers that everything that can be done to fill the prescriptions quickly is being accomplished. She has minimized additional delays and frustration for the customers by making sure they know where other departments are located. By calling them when the prescriptions are ready, she has demonstrated a respect for their time. The customers are impressed by Maria's concern for the inconvenience and offer to come back at a specified time, instead of Maria having to page them.

Stressful situations can occur in all work environments. However, by their nature, hospitals tend to be more stressful than other work places. These situations can be eased by enlisting the assistance of coworkers. By directing your attention to the root of the problem, solutions can be reached.

Further Discussion

1. What would have happened if Maria had decided to keep the potential problems to herself and open for business as usual?

2. Some employees decide to blame the hospital they work for when there are problems meeting the needs of patients. How do you think the customers would have reacted if Maria chose to criticize Community Hospital instead of taking the positive actions described?

3. How do you feel when you have to wait for something you have ordered?

Effective Communication

"The art of conversation is the art of hearing as well as of being heard."
William Hazlitt, 1826

Communicating effectively means that you actively listen to what is being said. Listening is not a passive act. In order to understand the meaning of what is being said, the listener must be aware of more than just the spoken word. When you are taking direction on some activity, ask yourself if the information makes sense based on your previous training. Is it consistent with established policies and procedures? If not, ask further questions for clarification.

When you are talking with someone, observe their body language at the same time. Patients are given instructions by the pharmacist about their medication. They may also be given written information about their drugs. A customer may tell you he or she understands the directions for a medication, but you may see a look of confusion on his or her face. If this occurs, you must probe further to find out if the person really does understand. Here are some suggestions for questions to ask when you want to verify the person understands what they have been told.

- "You look to me like you have a question. Can I explain something again?"
- "Can you repeat those directions back to me?"
- "How have you handled this medication before?"
- "How is this different?"

Verifying that the patient understands medication directions is good customer service and a legal necessity. Under the law, patients are considered to be vulnerable during times of illness. Patients must be given the opportunity to receive special instructions from the pharmacist the first time they take a medication and anytime thereafter. Many pharmacies have special forms to fill out or boxes to check when customers pick up their prescriptions, to indicate they have received instruction, or to decline this service. Healthcare workers must take additional steps to ensure that communication has been understood. Getting in the habit of asking patients to repeat directions back to you is a good way to prevent errors in medication administration and avoid legal problems. Keep in mind the limits of your training. If you feel that the client has additional questions that require the help of the pharmacist, do not hesitate to request that assistance. Figure 3-2 illustrates the feedback loop in communication. Practice this process in daily conversation. To become skilled, it takes practice. If this seems like an unnecessary use of time, consider the following "In Real Life" scenario. Incidents like this really do happen!

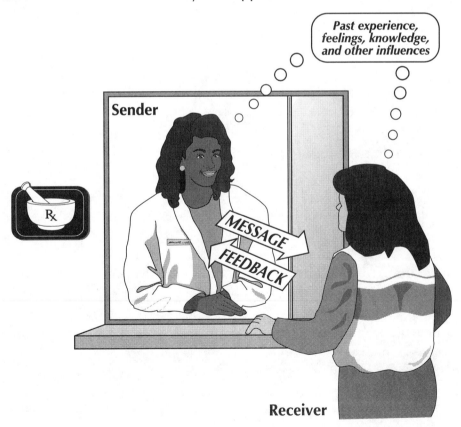

Figure 3-2: Each person in a conversation is affected by past experience, feelings, knowledge, and other influences, such as noise in the room.

In Real Life...

Mrs. Tran is a cancer patient undergoing **chemotherapy**. She was diagnosed with cancer several months ago. She is 81 years old. Mr. Tran is 82 years old. Although he is doing well for his age, his eyesight is failing. He is becoming more and more fatigued with his wife's care.

On this visit to the pharmacy, Mr. Tran is getting some new medication to control his wife's pain. He is also refilling a number of her usual prescriptions. One of the medications is morphine sulfate, a powerful **narcotic**, to be given **intramuscularly**. This is a new medication. She had previously been taking Tylenol® #3 (Tylenol® with a $^1/_2$ grain of codeine) in tablet form, for pain. Mr. Tran also obtains a number of bottles of sterile normal saline, for use in irrigating Mrs. Tran's special catheter used for her cancer medication.

Jeff is the pharmacy clerk at the cash register when Mr. Tran pays for his supplies. Because Mr. Tran's wife has been sick for a long time, Jeff knows him well. He waits on him almost every time Mr. Tran comes to the pharmacy. Jeff comments on the change in pain medication and asks Mr. Tran who had taught him to give his wife "shots." Mr. Tran proudly reports that the nurse in the doctor's office helps him. Jeff thinks that this is a lot of new medication for Mr. Tran to pick up for his wife all at one time, but decides it must be OK as the doctor is involved. Jeff lets Mr. Tran leave without any further explanation or questioning, even though he knows that the pharmacist must be called to consult with the customer when a new medication is prescribed.

In two days, Mrs. Tran is in the hospital again. Mr. Tran stops by the pharmacy to get some of his own medication filled while his wife is being taken care of by the hospital staff. Jeff is puzzled by Mrs. Tran's sudden readmission to the hospital. When Jeff questions Mr. Tran, he discovers that Mr. Tran had been injecting the normal saline, instead of the morphine sulfate, into his wife for pain control. Jeff realizes this because Mr. Tran mentions how much easier it is to handle the larger bottles (the normal saline bottles) than the smaller ones (the morphine bottles). Mrs. Tran had not received any morphine! Since Mrs. Tran's catheter was only irrigated once every two weeks, he had not given her any of the morphine yet!

---

narcotic: a drug that suppresses the central nervous system to relieve pain; can be habit-forming.

Jeff felt responsible for Mrs. Tran's hospitalization. In fact, several people are responsible for the misunderstanding. The physician, office nurse, and pharmacist all share in the problem. The best way to avoid blame is to prevent errors from happening. If you think a customer does not understand something about the medication, refer him or her to the pharmacist before the customer leaves the pharmacy! Going the extra mile for a customer will pay off in repeat business, enhance the pleasant atmosphere of the workplace, and most importantly, assure the quality of care every patient deserves.

Studies have shown the following behaviors indicate good customer service:

- Escorting customers to the shelf where an item is located.
- Smiling.
- Exhibiting a courteous attitude.
- Calling the customers by name.

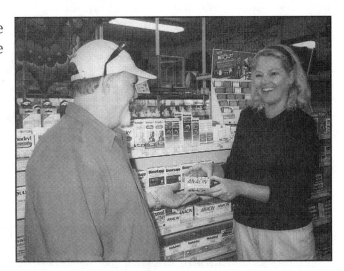

Figure 3-3: Good customer service is essential to a successful pharmacy.

Operating Business Machines in the Pharmacy

There are a number of machines in the pharmacy, whether hospital or retail, that a pharmacy clerk might have to learn to operate. Two of these machines are a cash register and a credit card scanner.

The Cash Register

A large part of the pharmacy clerk's day will be spent operating a cash register. It is important to master this skill first when going to a job in a retail pharmacy. There are a wide variety of cash registers, but the basic principles are the same.

First, most cash registers require electricity in order to operate. Many have digital displays and a pad of buttons and keys describing certain categories of products. There are also compartments for the register tape, the cash, and, in some instances, a separate compartment for checks and credit card receipts.

Many cash registers require that the user enter an identifying code before a transaction can be processed. Each employee is given a numeric code to be used for this purpose. The sale begins with inputting this code. The pharmacy clerk will enter the quantity, cost of medications being purchased, and the identifying code for the department or type of medication. For example, when a customer purchases a bottle of aspirin, a prescription for antibiotics, and some syringes, the pharmacy clerk would follow the procedure listed below.

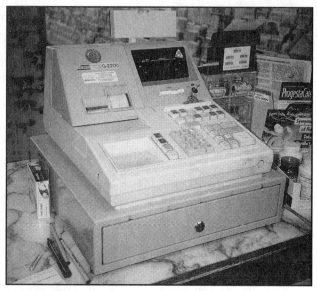

Figure 3-4: Computerized cash registers can serve as a backup for inventory control.

1. Begin by entering his or her code (eg, 321).

2. Press the number keys for $4.50 (the price of the aspirin).

3. Press the key for *OTC* (over-the-counter) medication since aspirin is not a prescription item.

4. Press *Enter* to process that item.

5. Press the number keys for $23.00 for the antibiotics and the department code for prescription medication.

6. Press *Enter* to process that item.

7. Press the number keys for $24.00 for the syringes and the department code for medical equipment.

8. Press *Enter* to process that item.

Once all the items are entered into the cash register, the *Subtotal* key is pressed. Then press the key to automatically add state and local taxes. In some states, no sales tax is charged on prescription medications or certain medical supplies. The final key pressed is the *Total* key. This usually tells the cash register to print a receipt. The cash drawer will open automatically and the money can be exchanged.

Cash registers with scanning features are common today. Less data entry is necessary as scanners feed information into a computer in a cash register. Bar codes are read from prescription labels and price tags on other merchandise. Bar codes are a series of black lines and spaces in a specified sequence that correspond to alphanumeric characters. These codes contain information such as the item number of the product, its price, and the department from which it came. The computer uses the information obtained from the bar code to recall previous information about the prescription, such as the number of refills that remain.

Figure 3-5: A Bar Code

You may find yourself working with a variety of cash registers during your career. It is always best to be oriented to the equipment you will use as soon as you obtain a job or new equipment arrives.

The Credit Card Scanner

Many customers use a credit card in the pharmacy. Credit card sales involve obtaining authorization for the purchase with a credit card company. Electronic scanning machines, many of which are built into or connected to a cash register, are in wide use for this purpose. These machines contact financial institutions via phone lines to electronically check the customer's credit line to verify the amount that can be added to the existing balance.

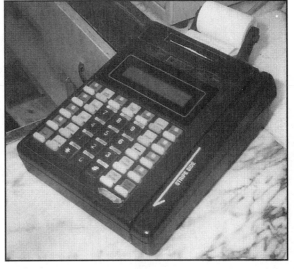

Figure 3-6: A Credit Card Scanner

To use a credit card scanner (methods may vary), slide the credit card through the scanner with the magnetic strip facing the side of the machine that reads the information. The machine will then prompt you for the amount of the purchase. After you enter the amount on the key pad, a message will show on the display screen that the machine is processing the transaction. This may take a few moments. The length of time varies depending on how busy the telephone lines are and how many other customers are trying to access the same system. Once an approval is given, an authorization number is provided. This number must be written on the charge slip. Sometimes a credit card scanner is not available, or is not connected to the cash register. In these cases, the transaction must be handled manually. The steps for completing a typical credit card charge manually are listed below.

1. Obtain the customer's credit card and check the expiration date.

2. Place the credit card in the machine to be imprinted.

3. Place the charge slip in the machine on top of the credit card.

4. Move the handle from left to right to imprint the charge card onto the slip.

5. Remove the credit card and the charge slip.

6. In the appropriate spaces on the charge slip, write this information:

    - your clerk ID number or initials.
    - a description of the items purchased.
    - the expiration date of the card. (Or verify the expiration date by circling or checking the appropriate box.)
    - the customer's phone number and/or ID number.

7. Obtain authorization for the purchase using an electronic system or the telephone.

8. Write the authorization number on the charge slip.

9. Have the customer sign the charge slip.

10. Destroy the carbon or give it to the customer.

11. Tear off the customer copy and give it and the credit card to the customer.

12. Place the credit receipts in the cash register.

If a customer is turned down by the financial institution that issued the credit card, the customer will have to contact that financial institution for more information. You will not be able to give the customer any information other than that the purchase was disallowed. There are strict confidentiality guidelines regarding credit information. Be pleasant and sympathetic to the customer. This is an embarrassing situation for the customer, and he or she will need to know you are trying to help as much as possible. Follow the directions of the credit card company representative about seizing a credit card that is reported stolen or is no longer valid.

If no electronic system for obtaining credit card information is available, you may be asked to call the credit card company. This is a simple matter that requires that you obtain the merchant number of your facility before you place the call. You also must have the amount of the purchase available, the credit card number, and the card's expiration date. Once you provide the credit card company with the correct information, you will generally get an approval number that must be written on the charge slip in the place provided. If the charge is denied, follow the guidelines in the previous paragraph for electronically declined credit card purchases. Figure 3-7 illustrates a completed credit card charge slip.

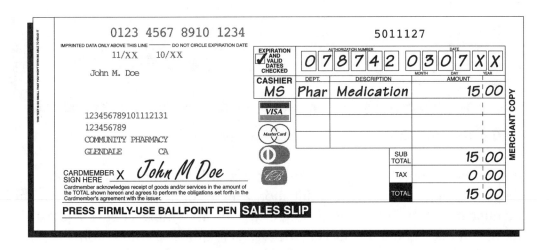

Figure 3-7: A Completed Credit Card Charge Slip

Accepting a Check for Payment

When you accept a check for reimbursement for medications or other supplies, you will need to verify that the information on the check is current and complete. For example, the customer's name and address must be imprinted on the check. Ask the customer if the address and telephone number on the check are current. If they are not, you will need to draw a line through the old information and write down the current information on the front of the check. The address and telephone number are the only items of information that can be changed on a properly imprinted check. The checking account number also must be imprinted on the check. Figure 3-8 illustrates a properly filled out check.

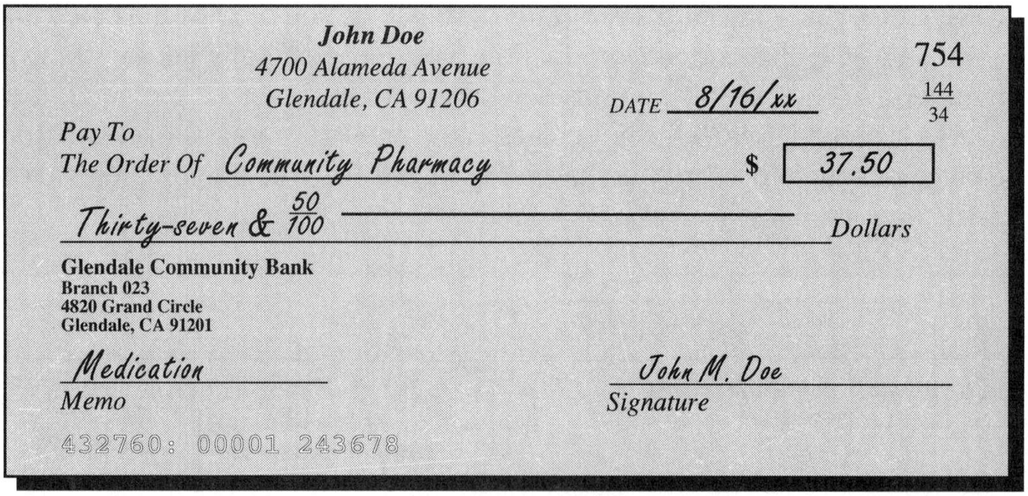

Figure 3-8: An Example of a Completed Check

Before you accept a check by putting it in the cash register, you will need to ask the customer for a piece of identification with his or her photograph on it. This identification ensures that the correct person is writing checks against the money in that account. A driver's license is the most common form of photo identification, but a military identification card or a state-issued identification card is acceptable as well. Check the name on the license and confirm that it is the same name that appears on the check. Look at both the check and the identification to make sure the signatures match. Often, you are expected to write the customer's driver's license number and its expiration date on the top of the face of the check.

Chapter Three • Essential Skills and Responsibilities

Verifying a check can be done relatively quickly, but should be done carefully. Customers who are honest will rarely mind that you check their identification. Try not to make your customers feel as if you suspect them of being dishonest. On rare occasions, a customer may grumble about having to show you identification. Simply explain to the customer that the procedure protects the person who holds the account by confirming that the proper person is using the checks. If you suspect that someone is using checks that do not belong to him or her, bring the situation to the attention of your supervisor. The vast majority of your customers will be honest, and their checks will be acceptable. In fact, you may never encounter a circumstance in which a customer tries to use a stolen check. But it pays to be careful, especially when you are dealing with **controlled substances**!

Insurance Plans and Drug Reimbursement

The inclusion of pharmacy benefits in an insurance policy is often seen as a real advantage by customers. Medications are becoming more and more costly. If the patient is left with little or no **copayment** on medications, the patient is more likely to take the medication the doctor prescribed. This is especially true of people who live on fixed incomes and have little money for expensive medications.

In years past, prescriptions were almost always paid directly by the patient at the time the prescription was filled. Now, reimbursement is often received from a **third-party payor**, such as a government program or a health insurance company. See Figure 3-9 for a list of insurance-related definitions.

However, pharmacy insurance benefits have led to complex methods of confirming eligibility for the pharmacy benefit when a customer comes in to purchase medication. The benefit to the pharmacy in accepting prepaid insurance plans is that there is a steady supply of customers. However, it requires a considerable amount of claims processing.

controlled substances: drugs defined and regulated by *The Controlled Substance Act of 1970* including narcotics, hallucinogens, depressants, and stimulants.

copayment: the share of medical costs for which the insured patient is responsible.

third-party payor: someone other than the patient who pays for prescription medications; third parties are usually government programs, insurance companies, or managed care plans, such as HMOs and PPOs.

Insurance Terms

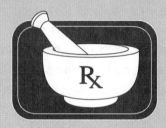

assignment of benefits	Payment of benefits made directly to the provider rather than to the patient.
capitation	A financial arrangement where a certain amount of money is received or paid out based on membership in the plan rather than on services rendered.
copayment	The money the patient/customer must pay each time a prescription is filled. This varies with each insurance policy and is usually a small amount of money.
deductible	An amount that must be paid by the patient or customer before the insurance company will pay any benefits. There are usually individual deductible amounts and a total amount for the family that must be met.
dependents	The individuals who are covered by an insurance policy through another person. (Usually a spouse and children.)
disenrollment	The process of terminating insurance coverage.
eligibility	Verification that a certain health service will be paid by the insurance company for a specific patient.
EPO	Exclusive provider organization. Similar to an HMO, but called exclusive because patients must stay within the network to receive the benefits of the plan.
gatekeeper	The term given to the primary care physician who must authorize care to be given by other providers except in real emergencies. A common requirement of HMOs.
healthcare provider	The physician, facility, or supplier that provides a medical service.

Figure 3-9A: Insurance Terms

Insurance Terms

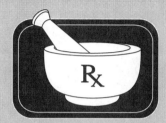

HMO — Health maintenance organization. A healthcare plan that provides care to enrolled members for a predetermined amount of money, usually prepaid on a per-member monthly basis. However, because of the increase in self-insured businesses and contracts with different financial arrangements, not all HMO plans require prepayment. Most utilize primary care physicians as gatekeepers, require preauthorization, and offer a limited panel of providers. Not all assume total financial risk so that some risk for medical expenses may be assumed by the providers.

insurance — A contract made between two people or two groups of people, in which one agrees to provide certain specified health benefits to the other.

insured — The individual who holds the policy.

IPA — Independent practice association. An organization that contracts first with a managed care plan and then with individual providers who agree to provide services at a reduced rate either by capitation or fee-for-service.

MCP — Managed care plan. Any system of healthcare management that incorporates ways to control costs through methods such as gatekeepers, preauthorization, panels of contracted providers, etc. Examples include HMO, IPA, PPO, and POS plans.

Medicaid/Medi-Cal — State provided health insurance for economically depressed individuals and families. **Coverage** is usually very specific and limited.

insured: an individual whose medical costs are covered, in part or wholly, by specific arrangements with an insurance company.

coverage: the amount and extent of financial responsibility. (ie, an insurance company may pay for a medication, but it will only pay for a specified dollar amount or a certain percentage).

Figure 3-9B: Insurance Terms (Cont.)

Insurance Terms

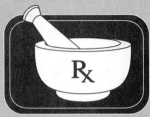

Medicare — Federal insurance provided to people over the age of 65, those who have permanent kidney failure, and people with certain disabilities. This is the fastest growing group of insured people. Coverage usually is very specific.

PCP — Primary care physician. A physician who serves as gatekeeper for a managed care plan. Usually a family practitioner, internist, pediatrician, or obstetrician/gynecologist who sees the patient first and then makes decisions as to whether to authorize care by other providers.

POS — Point of service. An arrangement where patients may receive care outside of their plan, but will receive reduced benefits and will have to pay more out of pocket.

PPO — Preferred provider organization. A plan in which patients can receive services from providers of their choice, but receive higher benefits if they go to providers contracted with the plan.

Universal Claim Form (UCF) — Paper form similar to a credit form. Used for manual processing of insurance claims when on-line claims processing (adjudication) is not possible.

Figure 3-9C: Insurance Terms (Cont.)

Establishing current eligibility for the pharmacy benefit is the most important step in the process of collecting payment. Even though a customer may have an unexpired insurance card, he or she may not be eligible for the insurance coverage. For instance, this may happen when a person leaves an employer and terminates the insurance. Also, employers sometimes change insurance companies. This would also make the person **ineligible** for the pharmacy benefit, despite the fact that he or she has a current insurance card.

ineligible: in a pharmacy, a term used to describe a person who is not allowed or not qualified to receive insurance benefits.

Some customers will have cards similar to automated teller cards. The most sophisticated of these cards have a magnetic strip that contains important information about the patient's medical history, as well as their insurance coverage. These cards may be updated automatically each time a new prescription is processed, allowing the pharmacist to monitor the patient's drug therapy more effectively. As a result, dangerous drug interactions or mixtures are avoided.

The more common insurance identification cards have the information necessary for insurance billing printed on them. The pharmacy staff enters the information from the card into the pharmacy computer system. For monitoring purposes, a **pharmacy patient profile** is created. Additional information about the patient's medical history must be obtained directly from the patient for this profile. See Chapter Six for more information on pharmacy patient profiles.

Another important consideration in processing third-party claims is whether or not the prescription itself is payable. Most insurance and government plans have a very specific **formulary**, or list of medications that are covered. If a drug is not listed on the plan's formulary, special permission may be needed to get the prescription reimbursed. Some companies refer to these as *treatment authorization requests* or as *non-formulary drug requests*.

formulary: a list of drugs for which an insurance company has agreed to provide partial or total reimbursement; a list of drugs that a hospital commonly stocks.

In addition, most third-party plans have quantity limits and restrictions on the frequency of dispensing. There may be a maximum number of doses that are permitted for each prescription – or the plan may require that a specific number of days supply of drug be dispensed. Most plans also have a maximum allowable ingredient cost for the drug itself, restricting the pharmacy to dispensing only certain brands of drug. Unless the prescription meets all of these criteria, the pharmacy will not receive reimbursement for dispensing the medication.

The vast majority of third-party prescription claims are processed on-line, giving the pharmacy immediate verification of the patient's eligibility. Any discrepancy in medication quantity or allowable cost will be transmitted directly to the pharmacy computer, so that the pharmacist can make necessary corrections. In most cases, the information received back from the third-party payor includes the co-pay amount to collect from the patient, as well as the amount that the pharmacy will receive as reimbursement from the insurance company or government program.

For the few third-party plans that do not use on-line claims processing, the pharmacy will have to complete and submit a manual claim form. Most often, the Universal Claim Form (UCF) is used for this purpose. Submitting claims manually is done as little as possible, since the pharmacy has no way of knowing whether the patient is truly eligible for prescription coverage or if the drug will be reimbursable in the quantity and brand dispensed.

In situations where the claim cannot be processed on-line, the pharmacy may have the patient sign a *waiver of liability*. By signing the waiver, the customer accepts responsibility for the bill if the third-party does not cover the cost of the prescription. This protects the pharmacy from losing revenue.

It is important to verify insurance coverage frequently—even on regular customers. When people change employers, their insurance coverage frequently changes as well. Insurance coverage can change for other reasons too. For instance, if a spouse obtains better coverage than that which is offered through the customer's own employer, the customer may switch over to the spouse's plan.

If a medication is not on a plan's formulary, or if on-line claims processing is not available for some reason, pharmacy policy may require that the pharmacy clerk call the third-party to get *prior authorization* for the prescription to be filled.

Chapter Three • Essential Skills and Responsibilities 3-23

The following checklist will help the pharmacy clerk to acquire the necessary information. In the case of a non-formulary request, the pharmacist or prescriber may need to provide the third-party with additional information before approval is granted.

- Get the telephone number of the insurance company and contact name (if any) from the customer.
- Get the customer's employer's name, customer's social security number, and the group number of the insurance policy.
- Obtain the insured's name if the customer is someone other than the insured, such as when a child is the patient.
- Call the company and tell them you are calling regarding eligibility.
- Give the insurance company the requested information.
- Get and record the insurance company representative's name and direct telephone number.
- Get any reference number or authorization number.
- Find out if there is any deductible or copayment, and if so the amount.
- Note the date and time the conversation with the representative occurred.

Often the verification can be done via touch-tone telephone, so the form may not always be necessary for more routine medications. But it will be helpful in more costly and unusual circumstances.

Insurance Verification Request

Name of Customer: _____ Phone: _____
Address: _____
Insurance Carrier: _____ Phone: _____
Address: _____
Plan Number: _____ Group Number: _____
Employer: _____

Insurance Information

Person Requesting Information: _____
Contact Name at Insurance Company: _____
Pharmacy Benefit: _____
_____

Maximum Reimbursement: _____
Generic/Brand: _____

Verification Number: _____

Billing Information

ATTN: _____
Address: _____
_____
_____
_____

Figure 3-10: An Insurance Verification Request

Chapter Three • Essential Skills and Responsibilities

In Real Life...

> A conversation to verify insurance coverage, between a pharmacy clerk (PC) and an insurance company representative (IR).
>
> PC: This is Rick Garcia calling for an eligibility check.
> IR: What is the insured's social security number?
> PC: 111-12-1234.
> IR: What is the insured's name?
> PC: Robert Morris, spelled M-o-r-r-i-s.
> IR: What is the patient's name and relationship to the insured?
> PC: Susan Morris, spouse.
> IR: Ms. Morris has a pharmacy benefit. This is a $1,000 maximum in prescription medication, which does not include medical equipment. There is a $5.00 copayment for each prescription ordered, and with each refill. Usual and customary rates apply. Each benefit year is 12 months from January through December.
> PC: Do you need any special information for billing?
> IR: No.
> PC: Are there any medications excluded from this plan?
> IR: Yes, any experimental drugs.
> PC: Are generic substitutes required?
> IR: Yes.
> PC: May I have your name and direct telephone number please?
> IR: My name is Sonia Arjuna, and my phone number is (123) 555-6043.
> PC: Is there an authorization number to use for billing?
> IR: No.
> PC: Thank you so much. Good-bye.

The customer may elect to pay for the prescription if the insurance company will not. Be sure to ask the customer about this option if the insurance company does not cover the medication. In some cases, the pharmacist might ask you to call the prescriber's office and let him or her know that the insurance company is denying coverage. Although the pharmacy clerk cannot request that another drug be prescribed, it is helpful to do all the preparatory work so that the pharmacist can get the medication changed.

Receipts can be very important in obtaining insurance reimbursement for prescriptions. Some people will choose to pay for their prescription and send the bill into their insurance company themselves. In some cases, the insurance company will require this and will generally reimburse the patient for a percentage of the cost of the medication. A regular tape (paper) receipt from a cash register is usually not enough documentation for the patient to obtain reimbursement. A special type of receipt that contains the name of the drug, its strength, etc., is given to the patient along with the cash register tape for the patient to submit to his or her insurance company for reimbursement. If a credit card is used, a copy of that sales slip is also given to the patient. Ask the customer if he or she needs a receipt and review it with the customer for completeness.

In some instances, the insurance carrier will also request the diagnosis that is being treated. This may require a telephone call to the physician who prescribed the medication. It may also be listed on the customer's bill or receipt from the physician. Receipts are also important in claiming medical expenses for income tax purposes. Be sure to provide receipts with every purchase.

Avoiding Cross-Contamination

cross-contamination: the making of a clean object or person unclean by contact with another object or person.

hygiene: cleanliness.

Cleanliness in the pharmacy is essential. Keeping both the pharmacy work areas and yourself clean will prevent **cross-contamination** from occurring. It also means that medications will be pure when dispensed. Handwashing is the single most important method of maintaining proper **hygiene**. Each pharmacy will have a designated place for handwashing. Special cleaning solutions may be used in some facilities. See the procedure on the following page.

Rubber or latex gloves should be used by pharmacy clerks when handling items that are potentially contaminated. Remember, gloves are no substitute for handwashing. It is still necessary to wash hands between jobs, after using the rest room, and after every contamination.

Figure 3-11: A neat and clean appearance is a MUST for anyone working in healthcare.

Chapter Three • Essential Skills and Responsibilities

Handwashing Technique

Materials needed:
- ✓ liquid soap
- ✓ dry paper towels
- ✓ cuticle stick or nail brush

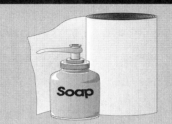

1. **Procedural Step:** Turn on the faucet. Adjust the temperature of the water to warm—don't burn yourself!
   Reason: Warmer water helps remove pathogens.

2. **Procedural Step:** Always wet your hands with the fingertips pointing down into, but not touching, the sink.
   Reason: Keeping your hands down keeps your forearms dry and prevents contaminated water on your forearms from running over your clean hands. (In most cases, your hands will be dirtier than your arms anyway, so concentrate on getting your hands clean.)

3. **Procedural Step:** Use a liberal amount of soap and rub the palms of your hands together several times.
   Reason: This friction will create a lather and help remove any unwanted viruses or bacteria from the skin surface.

4. **Procedural Step:** Put the palm of one hand over the back of the other hand and briskly rub them together.
   Reason: All parts of the hands are capable of carrying germs.

5. **Procedural Step:** Repeat step #4 using the opposite hands.
   Reason: To clean the other hand.

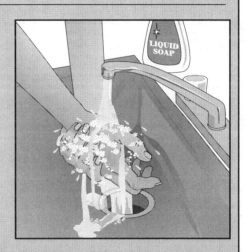

6. **Procedural Step:** Interlock the fingers of both hands and vigorously rub them together. You should scrub your hands for a total of two minutes.
   Reason: To remove harmful germs.

7. **Procedural Step:** Use an orange (cuticle) stick to clean under each nail. If a cuticle stick is not available, use a nail brush.
   Reason: To remove germs from under the nails.

8. **Procedural Step:** Rinse all soapy lather from the wrists and hands, continuing to point the hands downward.
   Reason: To prevent contaminated water on your forearms from running over your clean hands.

Handwashing Technique (Cont.)

9. **Procedural Step:** Leave the water running and dry all areas of the hands using a paper towel.
   Reason: Paper towels are disposable and prevent the spread of germs.

10. **Procedural Step:** Dispose of the wet paper towel. Obtain another paper towel and, placing the paper towel on the faucet handles, turn off the water. Make sure the towel is dry.
    Reason: A wet paper towel allows microorganisms to pass through the towel and back onto your clean hands. The dry paper towel will shield your hands from germs on the faucet. THE FAUCET AND SINK ALWAYS ARE CONSIDERED TO BE CONTAMINATED.

11. **Procedural Step:** Discard all debris and leave the sink and surrounding area clean, taking care not to recontaminate your hands.
    Reason: The area must be ready for the next person who wants to wash.

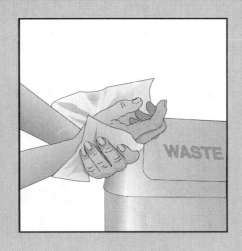

Well-kept hair and nails are also important for good hygiene; they should be kept neat and clean at all times. These requirements extend to clothes as well. Proper attire for the pharmacy clerk will vary from facility to facility, especially between clinical and retail settings. In all cases, dress codes will be dictated by the employer and may range from street clothes, to a smock, to a lab coat. It is important that these are clean and pressed also.

Cleaning the pharmacy's work surfaces properly is very important. Maintaining clean counters and mixing areas helps the pharmacist perform his or her work quickly and properly. Each facility will have its own procedures that will specify who is assigned to cleaning duty, and when and how the cleaning will be done. If you are not assigned the primary duty for cleaning an area, it is still important to do your share and clean up spills as they occur.

Contamination of Medications

If you are working with medications and they become contaminated, be sure to dispose of them properly. Items can be dropped on the floor, have liquid spilled on them, or be damaged in some other way. Each pharmacy will have a specific method of disposing of these medications, and you must be sure to use it. If the medication is a controlled substance, LET THE PHARMACIST KNOW it was contaminated and follow his or her instructions for proper disposal. These medications are carefully counted, and each one must be documented.

Needle Disposal

If syringes are used to mix medications or if you find a syringe on a counter, it should be disposed of in a **sharps container** (Figure 3-12). State and federal laws regulate the method of disposal for sharps containers. Do not look through these containers for lost articles as you could stick or cut yourself. Keep trash other than sharps out of these containers. For your protection and the protection of the people you work with, NEVER throw syringes in a trash can!

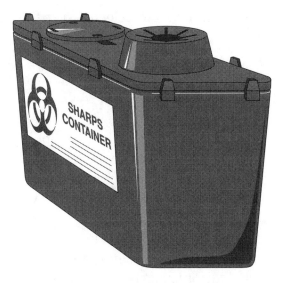

Figure 3-12: A Sharps Container

sharps container: a plastic container, usually red, that is designed for the safe disposal of used sharps.

Great care must be taken to minimize the risk of a needle stick. If a needle is improperly discarded in a trash receptacle that is not safe for sharps, employees could be stuck accidentally when disposing of trash. Many diseases, including AIDS, hepatitis, and other infections, can be transmitted via contaminated needles. However, in the pharmacy, the needles have been used for mixing medications, not for administering medications. Thus, they should not present the risk of contamination from blood-borne pathogens.

Committee Assignments

The larger the organization you work for, the greater the chance you will be assigned duties beyond your work in the pharmacy. Health systems generally have many committees that are designed to keep the organization current with standards of care in the community. A liaison committee with other pharmacies in the system is an example. There are also committees that assist the facility in meeting **accreditation** requirements, such as the safety committee. Other committees review forms, new products, and employee recreation activities. Committee work is an important way for the pharmacy clerk to contribute to the entire organization. Ask your supervisor about the committees and find out how new members are selected. Let the committee chairpersons know you are interested.

Chapter Summary

Although computers and technology are drastically reshaping pharmacy practice, customer service remains the foundation of a successful pharmacy. As a pharmacy clerk, you will be the customer's primary contact. Providing excellent customer service allows you to help assure your pharmacy's success.

Being a good pharmacy clerk requires that you master skills in several important areas: handling business machine transactions; communicating effectively with customers and co-workers; processing third-party reimbursements; and maintaining the cleanliness and safety of the your workplace. The duties performed by pharmacy clerks are challenging. With training and practice, you will become proficient — and you will provide valuable services to your customers and your employer.

Chapter Three • Essential Skills and Responsibilities   3-31

Name _____

Date _____

Student Enrichment Activities

Fill in the blanks for the following statements.

1. Needles are to be disposed of in _____ containers.

2. _____ is a word that means that the customer has been confirmed as eligible for insurance payment.

3. _____ is the single most important method of maintaining proper hygiene.

4. A waiver of liability is a form that_____
   _____
   _____.

5. A government program or insurance company that pays for a patient's prescription is called a _____ _____ _____.

6. Effective communication may include observing _____ _____.

7. A(n) _____ is the amount of money a customer must pay in addition to what the insurance company will pay.

8. A(n) _____ is a patient who receives treatment from a healthcare facility without being admitted to a hospital.

Match the words in Column A with the appropriate description in Column B.

Column A

9. _____ a good way to make sure directions are understood

10. _____ begins with the first words spoken to the patient, physician, or healthcare worker

11. _____ a way to make sure a medication is covered by insurance for reimbursement

12. _____ a series of lines, imprinted on products, that define price and product identification numbers

13. _____ a drug that suppresses the central nervous system

14. _____ contaminated

15. _____ has not met insurance company requirements for coverage

16. _____ avoids disconnecting a telephone call

17. _____ a list of drugs for which an insurance company has agreed to provide partial or total reimbursement; a list of drugs that a hospital commonly stocks

18. _____ often tells more about how a person feels than what they say

Column B

A. unclean
B. hold button
C. body language
D. have the customer repeat them back
E. narcotic
F. bar codes
G. formulary
H. ineligible
I. prior authorization request
J. customer service

Chapter Three • Essential Skills and Responsibilities   3-33

Name _____

Date _____

19. Describe aspects of the feedback loop in communication.

_____
_____
_____
_____
_____
_____

20. Describe a properly filled out check.

_____
_____
_____

21. Describe the procedure for credit card charges.

_____
_____
_____

22. What is a controlled substance?

_____
_____

Chapter Four
Pharmacology Basics

Objectives

After completing this chapter, you should be able to do the following:

1. Define and correctly spell each of the key terms.

2. List the common abbreviations used for dosage forms and routes of administration.

3. Explain the difference between generic, trade, and chemical naming of drugs.

4. Identify several reference textbooks used in the pharmacy.

5. List the major categories of medications and the primary forms in which medications are supplied.

6. List common drugs and why they are ordered.

Key Terms

- adverse drug reactions
- aerosol
- bioavailability
- chemical name
- Controlled Substances Act of 1970
- drug
- Drug Enforcement Administration (DEA)
- elixir
- emulsion
- generic equivalent
- generic name
- injectable
- lozenge
- pharmacokinetics
- side effects
- suppository
- trade name

Introduction

Working in the pharmacy becomes more meaningful when you have a basic understanding of the medications that are being dispensed. This chapter will explain what a "drug" is and describe how new drugs reach the market, how drugs are classified, and the dosage forms in which drugs are provided. In addition, the major pharmacologic categories will be listed, with examples of the most common drugs in each category.

Drugs and Their Development

drug: a chemical substance used to diagnose, prevent, or treat disease.

What is a **drug**? Most simply, a drug is a chemical. It can be used to prevent someone from getting sick, to diagnose an illness, to treat a symptom, or actually cure a disease. Drugs can be derived from plants, from animals, and by chemical **synthesis**. Substances that the human body makes can also be **replicated** and used as drugs.

Drugs have been around almost as long as human beings. For thousands of years, people have been treated with medicinal drugs derived from herbs and plants. Commonly used drugs that were originally extracted from plants include aspirin, codeine, and digitalis.

Today, the drug industry continues to develop new and improved drugs, creating unique chemicals in their research labs. However, new drug compounds are still being discovered in plants and from animal sources. Genetic engineering, which uses bacteria to reproduce chemicals such as "human" insulin and "human" growth hormone, has expanded the arsenal of available drugs.

New drugs go through an extensive series of tests before they can be sold to the public. When a new chemical compound is discovered, researchers perform simple laboratory tests to determine if the chemical has any potential use as a drug. If it does, the chemical will then undergo testing on animals. Human testing, called *clinical trials*, will begin only after the chemical has been thoroughly tested on animals. During clinical trials, the drug will be tested on both healthy volunteers and patients with the disorder that the drug is intended to treat. Very detailed records will be kept of each step in the testing process.

Before it can be sold in the United States, a drug must have the approval of the Food and Drug Administration (FDA). For all new drugs, the FDA must be satisfied that the drug is both *safe* and *effective*. Even after a drug is released, the FDA will continue to collect data on the drug's use through a program of *post-marketing surveillance*. In rare cases, a drug may be found to be harmful only after it is in widespread public use. Then the FDA can ask that the drug be withdrawn from the market.

Research and development of each new drug requires many years and many millions of dollars to complete. To protect the financial interests of the drug company that has discovered and tested a new drug, a *patent* is issued. The patent, which is based on the chemical structure of the drug, grants the drug manufacturer the exclusive rights to market that drug for between 17 and 22 years.

After the patent expires, other drug manufacturers can request FDA approval to sell the drug as a **generic equivalent**. Since the drug itself has already been proven to be safe and effective, the other companies do not need to repeat that research. However, they must prove to the FDA that their product is a *chemical duplicate* of the original drug. They must also prove that their product is *bioequivalent*, which means it has the same **bioavailability** as the original drug. This should guarantee that a patient can be treated as effectively with a generic equivalent as with the original drug.

generic equivalent: a drug with the same chemical structure and bioavailability as a trade name product.

bioavailability: the rate and extent of absorption of a drug into the bloodstream.

Generic equivalents frequently cost less than the original drug, since the generic manufacturers have not invested as much money in research and development as the original drug company. Many generic manufacturers do not advertise their products, which also reduces the cost of their products.

The trend toward cost containment has significantly increased the use of generic equivalents. Many insurance companies will reimburse only for prescriptions filled with generic medications. The FDA insists that there is no difference between the therapeutic action of trade name drugs and their generic equivalents. However, there is some controversy on the subject. Customers with questions about the effectiveness of generic medications should be directed to the pharmacist.

Drug Naming

chemical name: a drug name consisting of a formula that describes its chemical composition.

Drugs are referred to by three different names. Initially, a new drug is identified by its **chemical name**. The chemical name describes the exact chemical structure of the drug. It is meaningful to chemists working with the drug molecule, but is rarely used by healthcare workers or by the public.

generic name: the nonproprietary name of a drug, under which the drug is licensed and which is used by every manufacturer of that drug.

ALL drugs also have a common, or **generic name**. The generic name, which may be a simplified form of the chemical name, is the officially recognized name of that drug. Every company that manufactures a particular drug will use the *same* generic name to identify it. Even if a drug does not yet have a *generic equivalent*, it will still have a *generic name*. By law, the generic name of the drug must appear on each drug product label.

trade name: a drug name created by its manufacturer (ie, Coumadin® or Tylenol®) that may be protected by a trademark; a brand name.

Some drugs also have a *brand* name or **trade name**. The original manufacturer of a drug usually creates the trade name as a catchy, easy-to-remember name. This is important since trade names are often used in advertising drug products to prescribers and to the public. Trade names are capitalized and are protected as registered trademarks, as indicated by the symbol ® or ™. ONLY the drug company that owns the trademark is permitted to identify a drug by its trade name.

Remember that a drug *patent* protects the chemical structure of a drug. The *trademark* protects the drug's trade name. When other companies begin to produce generic equivalents of a drug, they are not permitted to use the same trade name. Some manufacturers of generic equivalents choose to create a new trade name for their brand of the drug. Most generic manufacturers do not create new trade names, however. They list *only* the drug's generic name on their product labels. When a manufacturer does list a trade name on a product label, the drug's generic name must also be listed.

Generic name:	ibuprofen
Trade names:	Motrin®, Nuprin®, Advil®
Chemical name:	(+) -2- (para-isobutylphenyl) propionic acid

Figure 4-1: Names for One Medication

Drug Salts

Many drug products are manufactured as chemical compounds, or "salts." This improves the drug's solubility and helps the body to absorb the drug. The additional chemical is usually listed after the drug's generic name, as in *flurazepam hydrochloride* or *flurazepam HCl*. Though the hydrochloride in this example doesn't have any therapeutic effect, it does affect the way the flurazepam is processed in the body. Changing the drug to a different salt might affect its **pharmacokinetics**.

Most prescribers do not specify the salt of the drug when ordering a medication. However, the product labels and many reference materials will show the complete generic name, including the chemical added to produce the salt. There are dozens of chemicals used to make drug salts. In addition to hydrochloride (HCl), the most common salts include:

- carbonate
- citrate
- gluconate
- hydroxide
- phosphate
- sodium
- sulfate

pharmacokinetics: the manner and rate by which the body absorbs, distributes, metabolizes, and eliminates a drug. Often referred to as "kinetics."

In some cases, a drug is available in more than one salt form. For example, Tofranil® contains imipramine *hydrochloride*, whereas Tofranil-PM® contains imipramine *pamoate*. Tofranil® and Tofranil-PM® would not be considered generic equivalents of each other. A generic equivalent must contain the same drug *in the same salt* as the medication ordered by the prescriber.

The salt of a drug can be very significant in certain conditions. Penicillin G, an antibiotic, is available in many injectable salts, including sodium, potassium, procaine, and benzathine. A prescriber might choose the *potassium* penicillin G for a patient with conditions like high blood pressure or congestive heart failure, since these patients must avoid *sodium*. The *procaine* and *benzathine* salts are suspensions, which are long-acting when injected into muscle tissue. If you have any doubt about whether the type of salt is important for a particular drug, ask the pharmacist.

Slang Names

There are many commonly used drugs that have slang or shortened nicknames. For instance, digoxin is often referred to as *dig* (pronounced "dij"). Epinephrine is often called *epi*. Nitroglycerin, a medication for chest pain, is frequently referred to as *nitro*. To avoid confusion, always verify the name of a medication by using its complete trade or generic name.

Drug Classifications

When the FDA evaluates the safety of a new drug product, they determine how safe that drug actually is. A drug that is safe enough to be taken without medical supervision is designated as a non-prescription drug. Non-prescription drugs are sold in many locations, from grocery stores to gas stations to hotel gift shops. Non-prescription drugs are often referred to as **OTC** drugs, since they can be sold "over-the-counter," without the need for a prescription. Even if OTC drugs are purchased in a pharmacy, they are seldom covered under a patient's health insurance plan.

Most new drugs do require medical supervision to assure the safety of the public. These drugs are determined to be "dangerous drugs," since they are not safe for self-administration by the patient. To restrict the use of these drugs, the FDA requires that they be dispensed only by prescription. Manufacturers of prescription drugs must show the federal "legend" on their product labels. The federal legend was recently simplified to the term: **Rx Only**. If this term does not appear on a product label, then that drug may be sold OTC.

Controlled Substances

Some medications have the potential for addiction or abuse. The vast majority of these drugs are prescription drugs, which are further identified as controlled substances. Although narcotics are the best-known controlled substances, stimulants (such as amphetamines and some weight-loss products), depressants (such as sedatives and anti-anxiety drugs), and hallucinogens are also classified as controlled substances.

The **Drug Enforcement Administration (DEA)** regulates the purchasing, prescribing, and dispensing of controlled substances. Prescribers and pharmacies are issued DEA numbers, which are used to track the flow of controlled substances from the manufacturer to the patient. This tracking system tightens the distribution network for these drugs, making **diversion** for illegal use more difficult. The DEA also attempts to reduce the risk of addiction, by putting restrictions on legitimate prescriptions for controlled substances.

Under the **Controlled Substances Act of 1970**, five categories of controlled substance drugs were created. These categories, called *schedules*, are designated by Roman numerals. Drugs are assigned to a schedule based upon the degree of their actual or potential abuse. When abuse patterns change, the DEA can reclassify a drug into a different schedule.

- **Schedule I drugs** are highly addictive drugs that have no legal medical use in the United States. These drugs are not available by prescription, because they have not had their safety and effectiveness proven to the FDA. Examples include heroin, marijuana, and LSD.

- **Schedule II drugs** contain the most highly addictive drugs that are FDA approved. The ordering and handling procedures for drugs in this schedule are tightly restricted to prevent abuse, theft, and diversion. States may require special prescription forms for Schedule II drugs. Refills are not permitted on prescriptions for drugs in Schedule II. Examples of Schedule II drugs include morphine, Demerol®, Dexedrine®, Ritalin®, and cocaine.

- **Schedule III drugs** have less risk of addiction and abuse than those in Schedule II. Although ordering and handling restrictions exist, they are not as strict as for Schedule II. Refills are permitted for Schedule III drugs, up to a maximum of five times within 6 months. Examples of Schedule III drugs include Tylenol® #3, Vicodin®, Meridia®, Marinol®, and the anabolic steroids.

Drug Enforcement Administration (DEA): an agency of the federal government responsible for regulating the import and export of narcotics and other substances, the transport of such drugs across state lines, and drug trafficking.

Controlled Substances Act of 1970: a law enacted to control the distribution and use of drugs with the potential for abuse, such as narcotics (opiates and opium derivatives), hallucinogens, stimulants, and depressants.

- **Schedule IV drugs** have less risk of addiction and abuse than those in Schedule III, although refill limits are the same. All benzodiazepine drugs are listed in Schedule IV, including Xanax®, Ativan®, and Valium®. Other Schedule IV drugs include phenobarbital, Darvocet-N®, and chloral hydrate.
- **Schedule V drugs** have minimal potential for drug abuse. Medications in this schedule often contain small amounts of addictive drugs, in combination with nonaddictive drugs. Examples include Robitussin AC®, Lomotil®, and Poly-Histine CS®. In a few states, certain Schedule V drugs can be purchased without a prescription. In these states, patients must be over 18 and must sign a registry book in order to purchase the drugs OTC.

It is impossible to memorize all of the different drugs in each controlled substance category. When in doubt, look at the label on the drug product or the listing in a pharmacy reference. Controlled substance categories are identified with a capital "C," with the Roman numeral of the schedule inside the "C." If that symbol is not shown on the label or in the listing, the drug is not a controlled substance.

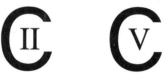

Figure 4-2: Examples of Controlled Substance Symbols

Chapter Four • Pharmacology Basics

Routes of Administration

Medications can be given to a patient by a number of methods, called **routes of administration**. The three basic routes of administration are:

- oral (by mouth)
- topical (including rectal administration and inhalation)
- injectable

The most common route of administration for drugs is the oral route. Drugs that are given orally are placed in the mouth and either swallowed or dissolved. The drug is then absorbed into the bloodstream and circulates to the spot where it is needed.

The choice of route depends primarily on the patient's condition. For example, an unconscious patient could not swallow an oral medication, so the rectal or injectable route might be used as an alternative. These alternative routes could also be used in a nauseated patient, who might have difficulty keeping an oral medication in his or her stomach.

Some drugs can be given by only one route. Others can be given by many different routes. Additional information on the routes of administration is included in the following description of drug dosage forms.

Abbreviations: The Route of Administration

AD	right ear	**OU**	each eye (both eyes)
AS	left ear		
AU	each ear (both ears)	**PO**	by mouth (orally)
		PR	rectally
ID	intradermal	**SQ, SubQ**	subcutaneously
IM	intramuscular	**SL**	sublingually (under the tongue)
IV	intravenous		
OD	right eye	**TOP**	topically
OS	left eye		

Figure 4-3: Abbreviations for the Route of Medication Administration

Drug Dosage Forms

Medications come in a surprisingly wide variety of dosage forms. The selection of a dosage form is based upon the needs of the patient and the physical characteristics of the drug. Often a drug is available in more than one dosage form. This is especially true of medications that are used in both adults and children. For example, while most adults can swallow tablets or capsules, children may need flavored syrups or chewable tablets of their medications.

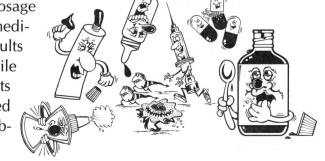

Oral Solids

Patients frequently refer to their oral solid medications as "pills." Historically, pills were handmade in the pharmacy, from a mixture of active and inactive ingredients. Pills were shaped into small balls or were rolled into long cylinders and sliced into disk-shaped pieces. True pills have not been made for decades, but patients still use that term when talking about their tablets and capsules.

Capsules are one of the most common oral solid dosage forms. Capsules are available in two basic types: hard-shell and soft- (or elastic) shell. Hard-shelled capsules consist of two halves of rigid gelatin that are filled with drug powder and fitted together. Some hard-shelled capsules are sealed with a band of gelatin to prevent the two halves from being pulled apart. Very few OTC drugs are available as hard-shelled capsules, because of the risk of product tampering.

Elastic capsules are made of thicker, pliable gelatin. The gelatin shell of an elastic capsule forms a hollow cylinder. The center of the elastic capsule is filled with drug in liquid form. These liquid-filled capsules are sometimes referred to as *liquid gelcaps* or as *liqui-gels*. Most patients prefer to take capsules, because their elongated shape makes them easy to swallow.

Tablets are another common oral solid. Tablets are made of powders compressed into shape by machine. Many tablets are round, although they can be of virtually any shape. Trade name drug manufacturers often create interestingly shaped tablets to distinguish their products from the generic equivalents. Tablets can also be shaped like capsules. This type of tablet is called a *caplet*.

Chapter Four • Pharmacology Basics 4-11

Patients may have trouble swallowing tablets due to their powdery surface and bad taste. To make the tablet easier to swallow, a coating may be added around the compressed core. A tablet coated with a layer of gelatin is called a *geltab*. *Gelcaps* are capsule-shaped tablets that are coated in gelatin. It is easy to mistake a gelcap for a true capsule, since the shape and surface look the same, but gelcaps have the solid center of a tablet.

Two other types of coating can be used to cover up the powder and mask the taste of a tablet: film coats and sugar coats. A film coat is a very thin layer of coating. It is often used on embossed tablets. Sugar coats are thicker, much like a candy coating. Sugar-coated tablets have caused problems when children have mistaken them for candy, resulting in drug overdoses.

Enteric coating is a very specialized type of coating, which is designed to dissolve only in the small intestines. Enteric coating is placed on drugs that can irritate the stomach, such as aspirin. Enteric coating is also used to protect drugs that might be destroyed by the stomach acids. In other words, enteric coats protect the stomach from the drug *or* protect the drug from the stomach.

Other tablet types are listed below:

- **Chewable** tablets, which must be chewed before they are swallowed. Chewable tablets are usually too large to swallow whole. Some chewables look more like cubes of candy than tablets. Adults as well as children use chewables.
- **Effervescent** tablets, which are dissolved in a full glass of water. The patient then drinks the water. Effervescent tablets should never be placed directly in the mouth.
- **Sublingual** tablets, which are tiny tablets placed under the tongue. Sublingual tablets provide an almost immediate effect.
- **Rapidly-disintegrating** tablets, which dissolve very quickly in the mouth. These tablets do not have to be swallowed, so they can be taken even if the patient doesn't have any water to drink.

lozenge:
solid medication administered by dissolving in the mouth.

Lozenges are the third type of oral solid. Sometimes called a *troche* (pronounced tro-key), this dosage form is like a piece of hard candy. Lozenges are held in the mouth until they dissolve, slowly releasing their drug content. Since lozenges are difficult for children to use, some manufacturers have created drug lollipops by putting sticks into lozenges.

Gums can also be used to deliver medications. As the patient chews a medicated gum, the drug dissolves in the patient's saliva and is swallowed.

Oral Liquids

Patients who cannot swallow oral solids rely on liquid dosage forms of medications. Young children, the elderly, and patients who have feeding tubes are candidates for liquid medications. The three broad categories of liquids used for drugs are solutions, suspensions, and emulsions. When used orally, these liquids are usually sweetened and flavored.

Solutions are liquids in which a drug powder has been dissolved. Oral solutions are usually aqueous (water-based). Because the drug has been completely dissolved, solutions are clear. There is usually no need to shake a solution. Specialized types of oral solutions include:

- **syrups**, which are sweetened with sugar, and
- **elixirs**, which use an alcohol and water mixture to dissolve the drug.

elixir:
an oral dosage form prepared by combining one or more drugs with a mixture of water, alcohol, sweeteners, and flavors.

Suspensions contain drug powders that have not been dissolved. Instead, the drug powder floats throughout the liquid portion of the suspension, making the product appear to be cloudy. Because the drug powder will eventually sink to the bottom of the container, suspensions must be shaken thoroughly before they are administered. Prescriptions for suspensions must carry an auxiliary label reminding the patient to "Shake Well Before Using."

emulsion:
a combination of two liquids that, though mixed, will not dissolve into one another (ie, oil and water).

Emulsions are formed by combining an aqueous liquid with an oil. Oil and water do not naturally mix, so an emulsifying agent is added to keep the emulsion from separating into layers. If it does, the emulsion has "cracked" and should be discarded.

Chapter Four • Pharmacology Basics 4-13

Abbreviations: Dosage Forms

cap	capsule	**susp**	suspension
cr	cream	**supp**	suppository
el, elix	elixir	**tab**	tablet
gtt	drop	**tr, tinct**	tincture
liq	liquid	**ung**	ointment
sol, soln	solution		

Figure 4-4: Abbreviations for the Dosage Forms

Topical Dosage Forms

Topical dosage forms are applied to body surfaces or inserted into body cavities. Many topical drugs have a local effect, although some are absorbed into the bloodstream and circulate throughout the body. Topicals that are absorbed have a higher risk of side effects than topicals that act locally.

Prescriptions for topicals should carry an auxiliary label to warn the patient that the drug is "For External Use Only." In addition, an auxiliary label may be needed to reinforce to the patient that the drug is "For the Eye" or "For the Ear."

Solutions, suspensions, and emulsions can all be used topically as well as orally. Unlike the oral forms, the topicals are not sweetened or flavored.

Topical solutions are administered as:

- enemas
- vaginal douches
- eyewashes
- eye *(ophthalmic)* and ear *(otic)* drops
- nose drops and nasal sprays
- inhalants

Topical suspensions must all be shaken before use. They include:

aerosol:
a substance suspended in a pressurized gas and administered as a mist, such as asthma medication or throat sprays.

- **aerosols**, which are used as topical sprays or in asthma inhalers, and
- **lotions**, which are spread on the skin surface.

Semi-solid topical dosage forms are also spread across the skin surface. Sterile versions of these dosage forms can be used as ophthalmics and placed inside the lower eyelid. Semi-solid dosage forms include:

- **creams**, which absorb readily into the skin. Most patients prefer creams because they are water-washable.
- **ointments**, which leave a greasy texture on the skin surface. Ointments do not wash off in plain water, so they may provide better protection for the skin.

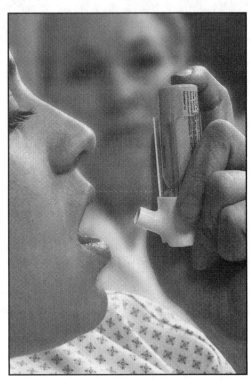

Figure 4-5: An inhaler dispenses aerosol medication.

Powders are solids that have been ground into tiny particles. Powders can be sprinkled onto the body or puffed into body cavities, such as the ear canal.

suppository:
semi-solid medication administered by melting or dissolving in the rectum, vagina, or urethra.

Suppositories are cones or cylinders of a drug that melt or dissolve when inserted into a body cavity. Suppositories are designed for insertion into the rectum, vagina, or urethra. Frequently supplied in foil wrappers, suppositories must be protected from excessive heat.

Transdermal patches look like small adhesive bandages. When applied to the body, transdermal patches release drugs into the bloodstream at a slow, constant rate. Patients who use transdermals generally have a good response to their medications, since they do not forget to take doses.

Chapter Four • Pharmacology Basics

Injectables

Medications can also be injected into the body by a variety of routes. To be given by injection, a drug must be in liquid form and must be sterile. There are several routes of **injectables**: intravenous, intramuscular, subcutaneous, and intradermal.

injectable: generally describes medications that can be administered by using a needle.

Intravenous (IV) medications enter the bloodstream directly through a catheter or needle placed in a vein. Solutions and emulsions are dosage forms that can be given intravenously. Suspensions cannot be given IV because the particles of undissolved drug powder would harm the patient.

Intramuscular (IM) medications are injected into muscle tissue where they slowly absorb into the bloodstream. Solutions and suspensions can be given IM.

Subcutaneous (SC or subQ) medications are injected into the fat layer just below the skin. The subcutaneous route is frequently used by patients who must inject medications (such as insulin) at home.

Intradermal (ID) injections, which place the drug into the skin layer, are most commonly used for skin tests.

Dosages

Drugs vary widely in the dosages in which they are prescribed. To be effective, a drug must be given in a high enough dose to produce the desired response. However, if too much drug is given, the patient can become toxic. Toxicity reactions are dangerous for the patient and may cause permanent damage to the body.

It is important to realize that drugs are given in varying amounts depending on the following considerations:

- **Age:** Infants and the elderly often receive lower doses of medications because their body systems are not fully functional.
- **Body weight:** The less a patient weighs, the less medication they are likely to need. For this reason, children receive smaller doses than adults. Very potent drugs are dosed on accurate measurements of a patient's daily weight.
- **Body composition:** Even if two patients weigh exactly the same amount, their drug doses may be different. This is because drugs accumulate in different body tissues. The balance of fat tissue to muscle tissue determines the dose of some drugs.

- **Gender:** In general, women have a higher percentage of body fat than men, so their body composition affects their drug dosages. In addition, the hormone differences in men and women may change the way their bodies handle drugs.
- **Disease states:** Liver, kidney, and circulatory diseases all can alter the way the body processes medications. When these diseases exist, it is often necessary to reduce the amount of medication prescribed.
- **Sensitivity:** Some patients are unusually sensitive to certain drugs and may require smaller doses to prevent uncomfortable or dangerous side effects.
- **Tolerance:** Patients may develop a tolerance for medications like narcotics and nasal sprays. In these cases, the patient needs higher doses to produce the desired effect from the drug.

It isn't unusual for patients to receive prescriptions for increasing doses of medication. For safety reasons, many prescribers start their patients on the lowest dose of a new prescription and gradually build the dose until the patient gets a good response. The pharmacist will monitor these dosage changes to make sure that the patient isn't taking two dosages of the same drug.

Drug manufacturers produce their products in the dosage sizes that are most often prescribed. There are so many drugs and so many dosages that they are impossible to memorize. As a rule of thumb, any dose that requires *more than two* or *less than half* of a tablet, capsule, or teaspoonful should be questioned.

Dosages may also vary within the same prescription. Sometimes the directions on a prescription will allow a patient to **titrate** the dose to a specific symptom. For example, a prescription for an analgesic may allow the patient to take *one or two tablets*, depending on how severe the pain is.

Interactions between drugs can also affect their dosages. When taken together, some drugs have a **synergistic** effect. With a synergistic effect, one or both of the drugs gets a boost in its activity, so that the patient may need to take a lower dose. An **antagonistic** effect has the opposite action. With an antagonistic effect, a drug partially blocks the effectiveness of another, so the dose may need to be increased. Pharmacists review all of a patient's medications to watch for these types of interactions. Most pharmacies have a computerized database of drug interactions to assist the pharmacist with monitoring for drug interactions.

Drug Effects

Every drug produces several different effects each time it is taken. A drug is prescribed for its **therapeutic effect**. Sometimes called a *pharmacologic effect*, the therapeutic effect is the reason the patient is taking the drug.

Even at normal doses, each drug will also have **side effects**. Side effects are unintentional, although most are not unexpected. While some side effects are beneficial, the harmful side effects are the ones that cause concern. These harmful side effects, or **adverse drug reactions**, can be mildly unpleasant for the patient (such as nausea), or they can be lethal (like bone marrow failure). Because side effects generally get worse as the dose of a drug is increased, patients are given the smallest effective dose of a drug.

Another drug effect is the **idiosyncratic reaction**. An idiosyncratic reaction is one in which the patient has an unusual or unpredictable response to a drug. For example, OTC antihistamines make most adults drowsy. A patient who gets jittery or has insomnia from an OTC antihistamine would be experiencing an idiosyncratic reaction.

Allergic reactions are another type of drug effect. When a patient experiences an allergic reaction, he or she may develop hives or some other type of rash. Allergic reactions can also cause the patient's lips and throat to swell, or the patient may have trouble breathing, like an asthma attack. Severe allergic reactions, such as anaphylactic shock, can even be fatal. If a patient calls the pharmacy to ask about symptoms that sound like an allergic reaction, immediately refer that call to the pharmacist.

For each medication that a patient takes, the risks of the possibly harmful effects must be weighed against the benefit of taking the drug (the therapeutic effect). Prescribers, pharmacists, and the patients themselves should assess this *risk versus benefit* relationship for all drugs, even OTCs.

---

side effect: an unintended reaction, such as headaches or nausea, resulting from the use of a medication.

adverse drug reactions: unfavorable and undesirable effects or toxicity in response to a pharmacological substance.

Drug Reference Materials

Because there are so many drugs available, most pharmacies will have a small library of drug reference books. These references are designed for healthcare professionals, so the language may be difficult to understand. Although customers may ask the pharmacy clerk about his or her medications, remember that drug information questions must be answered by the pharmacist.

Much of the drug information that the pharmacist needs is supplied by the manufacturers in the form of **package inserts**. These inserts, which are included with each package of drug product, contain all of the FDA-approved information about a drug product. Manufacturers provide the following information in a package insert:

- *Description:* chemical and physical composition of the drug.
- *Clinical Pharmacology:* what the drug does in the body; its therapeutic effects.
- *Indications and Usage:* the diseases or symptoms that the drug is used to treat.
- *Contraindications:* coexisting diseases or symptoms that increase the risk of taking the drug.
- *Warnings:* potential dangers associated with the use of the drug.
- *Precautions:* special circumstances that require a patient to use extra caution.
- *Adverse Reactions:* the harmful side effects that a patient might experience.
- *Overdosage:* the symptoms and treatment caused by excessive doses.
- *Dosage and Administration:* the appropriate dose of the medication and any special administration instructions.
- *How Supplied:* the dosage forms and strengths in which the drug is sold.

The package insert only contains information on the FDA-approved uses of a drug. If a drug is prescribed for an *off-label use,* that information will not be found in a package insert. The pharmacist will have to consult another more comprehensive reference book.

Chapter Four • Pharmacology Basics

4-19

The following reference books are usually available in the pharmacy:

- The *Physician's Desk Reference® (PDR®)* contains reprints of the package inserts of over 3000 medications, arranged by manufacturer and trade name. A very useful feature of the PDR is the Product Identification Guide, which presents full color, actual size photos of selected medications. There are separate PDR®s for herbal medicines and for non-prescription drugs and dietary supplements.

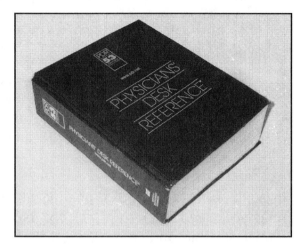

Figure 4-6: A Physician's Desk Reference

- The *American Drug Index (ADI)* is an alphabetical listing of drug products that is used like a dictionary. Information in the *ADI* is very brief, showing each drug's trade and generic names and its pharmacologic classification.

- The *American Hospital Formulary Service (AHFS®) Drug Information* is published by the American Society of Health-Systems Pharmacists. Used extensively in hospitals, this reference is considered to be unbiased and very comprehensive. Medications in this book are listed within their pharmacologic classifications, by their generic names.

- *Drug Facts and Comparisons®* also groups drugs by their pharmacologic classifications. One of the best features of this references is its charts, which allow a quick comparison of similar drug products. A loose-leaf version of this reference has monthly updates, so the information is very current.

- The *Drug Topics® Red Book®* is an extensive catalog of commercially-available prescription and OTC drugs, used primarily for pricing. The *Red Book®* contains a Product Identification section, with colored photos of selected drugs, and sections on pharmacy organizations and drug reimbursement information. The Clinical Reference Guide section provides lists of drug interactions, as well as lists of specialized drugs, such as sugar-free and alcohol-free products.

- The *United States Pharmacopeia Drug Information (USP-DI®)* is a three-volume set. One volume is *Advice for the Patient*, written in lay language. The other volumes contain more detailed drug information for the healthcare provider, including legal requirements for drug products.

- The *United States Pharmacopeia – National Formulary (USP-NF®)* contains the official standards for the production of drugs whose generic names are followed by the initials "USP." This reference is used primarily by drug manufacturers and may not be available in many pharmacies.

In addition to these books, pharmacies may have access to computerized reference materials. Many of the book references are also available in CD-ROM format or as an on-line resource. On-line resources, including the Internet, provide the most up-to-date reference information to both healthcare providers and the public. For example, the Food and Drug Administration (FDA), a government agency that provides food and drug information, offers a particularly good source of information on-line:

- Food and Drug Administration
  Internet address is: **http://www.fda.gov**

There are extensive references on this Internet site regarding how medications obtain approval. There is also specific information on how the rights of people involved in research studies are protected by the government. Additional information includes what the researchers investigating new sources and types of medication must do to apply for a research study, and the role of the FDA during the process. Many pharmaceutical manufacturers also have Internet sites. These can be easily accessed through an Internet search.

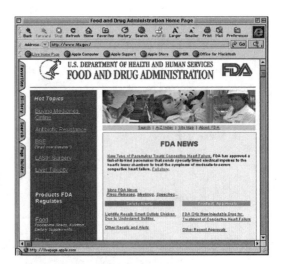

Figure 4-7: The Internet is a rich source of information about pharmacy issues.

Chapter Four • Pharmacology Basics

Pharmacologic Categories of Medication

A drug's action on the body determines its category. The following is a list of common categories, with examples of frequently used drugs in each class. The pharmacologic categories have been grouped by body system, so that the relationships of the drugs to their indications are more clear.

It is possible that a drug will be used for more than one indication. In that case, the drug will appear in more than one category.

Note that the generic names of some categories of drugs share common endings. This can serve as a memory device. Common endings are underlined to highlight their similarity.

Antimicrobials (Anti-infectives)

Used to prevent or treat infection by killing or stopping the growth of microorganisms.

Antibiotics are used for infections caused by bacteria. Examples:

Amoxil® (amoxicillin)
Augmentin® (amoxicillin/potassium clavulanate)
Bactrim® and Septra® (sulfamethoxazole with trimethoprim)
Bactroban® (mupirocin)
Biaxin® (clarithromycin)
Ceclor® (cefaclor)
Ceftin® (cefuroxime)
Cefzil® (cefprozil)
Cipro® (ciprofloxacin)
Cleocin T® (clindamycin topical)
Dynapen® (dicloxacillin)
Ery-Tab® (erythromycin)
Garamycin® (gentamicin)
Keflex® (cephalexin)
Levaquin® (levofloxacin)
Macrobid® (nitrofurantoin)
Neosporin® (neomycin, bacitracin, polymyxin)
Sumycin® (tetracycline)
Veetids® (penicillin VK)
Vibramycin® (doxycycline)
Zithromax® (azithromycin)

Antifungals are used for infections caused by fungus or yeast. Infections often involve the skin and nails, although fungi can also cause systemic (body-wide) infections. Examples:

amphotericin B
Diflucan® (fluconazole)
Fulvicin® and Grisactin® (griseofulvin)
Lamisil® (terbinafine)
Lotrimin® and Mycelex® (clotrimazole)
Monistat® (miconazole)
Nizoral® (ketoconazole)
nystatin
Sporanox® (itraconazole)
Terazol 7® (terconazole)

Antiseptics are used externally for handwashing or wound care. Examples:

Betadine® (povidone-iodine)
Hibiclens® (chlorhexidine)
pHisoHex® (hexachlorophene)

Antivirals are used for infections caused by viruses, such as influenza, herpes, and HIV. Antiviral drugs cannot cure a viral infection, but they do slow the progress of the infection or ease the symptoms. Examples:

Famvir® (famciclovir)
Foscavir® (foscarnet)
Symmetrel® (amantadine)
Valtrex® (valacyclovir)
Videx® (didanosine)
Vira-A® and Virazole® (ribavirin)
Zovirax® (acyclovir)

Antineoplastics

Antineoplastics are used in the treatment of cancer to control or minimize the growth of malignant tumor cells. Examples:

Cytoxan® (cyclophosphamide)
Efudex® (5-fluorouracil)
Leukeran® (chlorambucil)
Myleran® (busulfan)
Oncovin® (vincristine)
Velban® (vinblastine)

See additional listing under the Endocrine (Hormone) System Medications.

Electrolyte Replacements

Electrolytes are minerals dissolved in the bloodstream. The correct balance of electrolytes is necessary for the body to function properly. Potassium chloride (abbreviated as KCl) is the most commonly prescribed oral electrolyte replacement. Examples: K-Dur® and Klor-Con®.

Calcium supplements are also important electrolyte replacements. Examples:

Caltrate®
Os-Cal®
Viactiv®

Chapter Four • Pharmacology Basics

Cardiovascular System Medications

Antiarrhythmics regulate the rhythm of the heart's contractions. Examples:

Betapace (sotalol)
Cardizem® (diltiazem)
Cordarone® (amiodarone)
Inderal® (propranolol)

Isoptin® and Calan® (verapamil)
Pronestyl® and Procan® (procainamide)
Quinaglute® (quinidine)
Xylocaine® (lidocaine)

Anticoagulants, sometimes called "blood thinners," are used to control blood clotting. Examples:

Coumadin® (warfarin)
heparin

Lovenox® (enoxaparin)

Antihypertensives are used to treat hypertension (high blood pressure) by lowering blood pressure to the normal range. One of the most prescribed classifications in the United States, the antihypertensives fall into several sub-categories:

- *Angiotensin Converting Enzyme (ACE) Inhibitors*:

    Accupril® (quina<u>pril</u>)
    Altace® (rami<u>pril</u>)
    Capoten® (capto<u>pril</u>)
    Lotensin® (benaze<u>pril</u>)

    Monopril® (fosino<u>pril</u>)
    Prinivil® and Zestril® (lisino<u>pril</u>)
    Vasotec® (enala<u>pril</u>)

- *Angiotensin Receptor Blockers (ARBs)*:

    Cozaar® (lo<u>sartan</u>)

    Diovan® (val<u>sartan</u>)

- *Alpha-One Blockers*:

    Cardura® (dox<u>azosin</u>)
    Hytrin® (ter<u>azosin</u>)

    Minipress® (pr<u>azosin</u>)

- *Beta-Blockers*:

    Corgard® (nad<u>olol</u>)
    Inderal® (propran<u>olol</u>)

    Lopressor® (metop<u>rolol</u>)
    Tenormin® and Toprol XL® (aten<u>olol</u>)

- *Calcium Channel Blockers:*

    Cardizem® and Tiazac® (diltiazem)
    Isoptin® and Calan® (verapamil)
    Norvasc® (aml<u>odipine</u>)
    Plendil® (fel<u>odipine</u>)
    Procardia® and Adalat® (nife<u>dipine</u>)

- *Alpha-Two Agonists:*

    Aldomet® (methyldopa)
    Catapres® (clonidine)

Many combination products are also used to treat hypertension. By using two drugs together, better control is achieved. Most combination products for hypertension contain one of the drugs listed above, plus a diuretic. Examples:

Hyzaar®
Lotrel®
Prinzide®

Zestoretic®
Ziac®

Antihyperlipidemics, such as Lopid® (gemfibrozil) and Questran® (cholestyramine), are used to decrease cholesterol levels. The most-used group of antihyperlipidemics prevents the liver from making cholesterol. Examples:

Lescol® (flu<u>vastatin</u>)
Lipitor® (ator<u>vastatin</u>)
Mevacor® (lo<u>vastatin</u>)

Pravachol® (pra<u>vastatin</u>)
Zocor® (sim<u>vastatin</u>)

Cardiotonics stimulate the contraction of the heart muscle, which makes them useful in the treatment of heart failure. Example: Lanoxin® (digoxin).

Vasodilators relax blood vessels, which improves blood flow. The coronary vasodilators are used to treat angina (chest pain due to a lack of oxygen in heart muscle.) Examples of anti-anginal vasodilators:

Imdur® (isosorbide mononitrate)
Isordil® (isosorbide dinitrate)

Nitrostat® and Nitro-Dur® (nitroglycerin - abbreviated NTG)
Persantine® (dipyridamole)

Vasopressors contract blood vessels, which increases blood pressure. These drugs are used to treat patients in shock. Example: Intropin® (dopamine).

Chapter Four • Pharmacology Basics

Note that some cardiovascular drugs have actions that make them useful in treating several types of disease. Beta-blockers and calcium channel blockers are also used to control irregular heart rhythms. Some drugs in these two categories are also used to treat angina; they slow the heart so that it doesn't require as much oxygen.

Digestive System Medications

Antacids neutralize stomach acid to relieve occasional indigestion or heartburn. Examples:

Maalox® and Mylanta® (magnesium and aluminum hydroxides)
Riopan® (magaldrate)

Tums® (calcium carbonate)

Antidiarrheals slow movement in the intestines to reduce diarrhea. Examples:

Imodium® (loperamide)
Kaopectate® (attapulgite)

Lomotil® (diphenoxylate/atropine)
Pepto-Bismol® (bismuth subsalicylate)

Anti-Emetics control nausea and vomiting. Examples:

Antivert® and Bonine® (meclizine)
Compazine® (prochlorperazine)
Reglan® (metoclopramide)

Phenergan® (promethazine)
Tigan® (trimethobenzamide)
Zofran® (ondansetron)

Antiflatulents control gas, or flatus. Examples:

Gas-X® (simethicone)
Mylicon® (simethicone)

Phazyme® (simethicone)

Antispasmodics treat spasms by relaxing the smooth muscle in the stomach and intestines. Examples:

Bentyl® (dicyclomine)
Donnatal® (belladonna alkaloids and phenobarbital)

Pro-Banthine® (propantheline)

Emetics are used to cause vomiting in cases of accidental poisoning or drug overdose. Example: ipecac syrup.

Laxatives and *Stool Softeners* stimulate bowel movements to treat constipation. Examples:

Colace® (docusate sodium)
Dulcolax® (bisacodyl)
Metamucil® (psyllium)

milk of magnesia (abbreviated MOM; magnesium hydroxide)
Senokot® (senna)
Surfak® (docusate calcium)

Ulcer treatments include drugs that stop the stomach from producing acid. These drugs are also used to treat Gastroesophageal Reflux Disease (GERD), which causes chronic heartburn.

- *Histamine-2 (H-2) Antagonists:*

    Axid® (niza<u>tidine</u>)
    Pepcid® (famo<u>tidine</u>)
    Tagamet® (cime<u>tidine</u>)
    Zantac® (rani<u>tidine</u>)

- *Acid Pump Inhibitors* also called *Antisecretory Drugs:* Prevacid® (lanso<u>prazole</u>) and Prilosec® (ome<u>prazole</u>)

A more permanent cure for ulcers is achieved by using antibiotics in combination with the drugs above. Examples: Helidac® and Tritec®.

Endocrine (Hormone) System Medications

Androgens are male hormones, used to increase muscle mass (an anabolic effect) or to replace testosterone deficiencies. Examples:

Anadrol® (oxymetholone)
Androderm® (testosterone)

Oxandrin® (oxandrolone)

Antidiabetics are used in the treatment of diabetes. Many diabetics use oral medications to stimulate their production of insulin. Examples of oral medications:

Amaryl® (glimepiride)
DiaBeta® and Micronase® (glyburide)

Glucophage® (metformin)
Glucotrol® (glipizide)

Other diabetics must use injections of insulin or insulin-like substances. Examples:

Humalog®
Humulin®

Novolin®

Chapter Four • Pharmacology Basics

Antineoplastics are used in the treatment of certain types of tumors, particularly breast and prostate, that can be treated with hormones. Examples:

Casodex® (bicalutamide)
Cytadren® (aminoglutethimide)
Eulexin® (flutamide)
Lysodren® (mitotane)
Megace® (megestrol)
Nolvadex® (tamoxifen)

Corticosteroids, usually called "steroids," are used to decrease inflammation. Oral and injectable steroids are used for a variety of inflammatory conditions, such as dermatitis, arthritis, and lupus. Examples:

Aristocort® (triamcinolone)
Decadron® (dexamethasone)
Deltasone® (prednisone)
Medrol® and Solu-Medrol® (methylprednisolone)
Pediapred® (prednisolone)
Solu-Cortef® (hydrocortisone)

Topical steroids are used for skin disorders, from minor skin irritations to psoriasis. Examples:

hydrocortisone (abbreviated as HC)
Diprolene® (betamethasone)
Elocon® (mometasone)
Lidex® (fluocinonide)
Temovate® (clobetasol)
Topicort® (desoximetasone)

Steroids can be used by inhalation to prevent asthma attacks, or as nasal sprays to control the symptoms of allergic rhinitis (hay fever). Examples:

Aerobid® and Nasalide® (flunisolide)
Azmacort® and Nasacort® (triamcinolone)
Flonase® and Flovent® (fluticasone)
Nasonex® (mometasone)
Pulmicort® and Rhinocort® (budesonide)
Vancenase AQ® and Vanceril® (beclomethasone)

Estrogens and *Progestins* are used in the treatment of female reproductive disorders and menopause. Estrogens protect post-menopausal women from osteoporosis and certain cardiovascular diseases. Examples:

Climara® and Estraderm® (estradiol)
Estratab® (esterified estrogens)
Premarin® (conjugated estrogens)
Premphase® and Prempro® (conjugated estrogens with medroxyprogesterone)
Provera® and Cycrin® (medroxyprogesterone)

- *Contraceptives*: estrogens, usually ethinyl estradiol, and/or progestins used to prevent conception, or pregnancy. Most are tablets dispensed in dial-packs. Examples:

Alesse®	Ortho Tri-Cyclen®
Desogen®	Ortho-Novum®
Lo/Ovral®	Tri-Levlen®
Loestrin®	Triphasil®

  Norplant® (levonorgestrel) is a contraceptive that is implanted under the skin and slowly releases medication for months.

Osteoporosis Treatments are used to increase the bone density and prevent fractures, especially in post-menopausal women. Examples:

Evista® (raloxifene)	Miacalcin® (calcitonin)
Fosamax® (alendronate)	

Calcium supplements are also beneficial.

Thyroid Replacements are used in patients whose thyroid gland does not produce enough thyroid hormone. Examples:

Armour® thyroid	Levoxyl® and Synthroid® (levothyroxine)
Levothroid®	

Nervous System Medications

Analgesics are used to relieve pain.

- *Non-Narcotic Analgesics:* milder pain relieving medications that do not contain controlled substances. Examples:

aspirin	Ultram® (tramadol)
Tylenol® (acetaminophen)	

  See also the Non-Steroidal Anti-Inflammatory Drugs listed below.

- *Narcotic Agonist Analgesics:* controlled substances that treat moderate to severe pain. Examples:

codeine	Dilaudid® (hydromorphone)
morphine	Oxycontin® (oxycodone)
Demerol® (meperidine)	

Chapter Four • Pharmacology Basics

Analgesics also include combinations of narcotic with non-narcotic analgesics. Examples:

Darvocet-N® 100
Percocet®
Roxicet®
Tylenol® #3 (with codeine)
Tylox®
Vicodin®
Vicoprofen®

Anesthetics eliminate sensations.

- *General:* medications used to produce a comatose state for surgery. Examples:

  nitrous oxide, which is inhaled
  Brevital Sodium® (methohexital), given intravenously
  Diprivan® (propofol), given intravenously
  Pentothal® (thiopental), given intravenously

- *Local:* topical and injectable medications used to decrease sensations to a specific part of the body. Examples: Marcaine® (bupivacaine) and Xylocaine® (lidocaine).

Anticonvulsants, or *Anti-Epileptics*, are used to control seizures. Examples:

phenobarbital
Depakote® (divalproex sodium)
Dilantin® (phenytoin)
Klonopin® (clonazepam)
Neurontin® (gabapentin)
Tegretol® (carbamazepine)

Several drugs in this classification are used to treat nerve pain as well as bipolar disorder.

Antidepressants relieve depression. Examples:

Celexa® (citalopram)
Desyrel® (trazodone)
Effexor® (venlafaxine)
Elavil® (amitriptyline)
Paxil® (paroxetine)
Prozac® (fluoxetine)
Remeron® (mirtazapine)
Serzone® (nefazodone)
Sinequan® (doxepin)
Tofranil® (imipramine)
Wellbutrin® (bupropion)
Zoloft® (sertraline)

Zyban® is another brand of bupropion, which is used to help patients stop smoking.

Anxiolytics, or *Anti-Anxiety Drugs*, are minor tranquilizers, intended to calm patients and reduce their anxiety level. Many drugs in this class are benzodiazepines, as indicated by the "-azepam" or "-azolam" in their generic names. Examples:

Ativan® (lor<u>azepam</u>)
BuSpar® (buspirone)
Librium® (chlordiazepoxide)
Serax® (ox<u>azepam</u>)

Valium® (di<u>azepam</u>)
Vistaril® (hydroxyzine)
Xanax® (alpr<u>azolam</u>)

Antipsychotics are major tranquilizers, used to control the hallucinations and delusions that are common in psychosis. These drugs are also used to control severe agitation. Examples:

Haldol® (haloperidol)
Mellaril® (thioridazine)
Navane® (thiothixene)
Risperdal® (risperidone)

Thorazine® (chlorpromazine)
Stelazine® (trifluoperazine)
Zyprexa® (olanzapine)

Migraine Treatments relieve the pain of migraine headaches. Examples: Imitrex® (suma<u>triptan</u>) and Zomig (zolmi<u>triptan</u>). NSAIDs and analgesics are also used to treat migraines.

Sedative/Hypnotics are used for the short-term treatment of sleep disorders, such as insomnia. Some of these drugs are also benzodiazepines. Examples:

Ambien® (zolpidem)
Dalmane® (flur<u>azepam</u>)
Halcion® (tri<u>azolam</u>)

Noctec® (chloral hydrate)
Restoril® (tem<u>azepam</u>)

OTC products for sleep frequently contain diphenhydramine (same as Benadryl®) or doxylamine (in Unisom®).

Stimulants are used primarily to treat Attention Deficit Disorder. Examples: Adderall® (amphetamine combination) and Ritalin® (methylphenidate).

Chapter Four • Pharmacology Basics

Musculoskeletal System Medications

Non-Steroidal Anti-Inflammatory Drugs (NSAIDs) are used to treat inflammation of the joints and other musculoskeletal structures. NSAIDs, which are effective pain and fever reducers, do not have the severe side effects associated with the anti-inflammatory steroids. Examples:

Celebrex® (celecoxib)
Clinoril® (sulindac)
Daypro® (oxaprozin)
Feldene® (piroxicam)
Indocin® (indomethacin)
Lodine® (etodolac)

Motrin® (ibuprofen)
Naprosyn® (naproxen)
Relafen® (nabumetone)
Toradol® (ketorolac)
Vioxx® (rofecoxib)
Voltaren® (diclofenac)

Skeletal Muscle Relaxants relax muscle spasms caused by overuse or injury. Examples:

Flexeril® (cyclobenzaprine)
Lioresal® (baclofen)
Paraflex® (chlorzoxazone)

Robaxin® (methocarbamol)
Skelaxin® (metaxalone)
Soma® (carisoprodol)

Respiratory System Medications

Antihistamines control the symptoms of allergy and colds, such as itchy eyes and runny noses. Examples:

Allegra® (fexofenadine)
Atarax® and Vistaril® (hydroxyzine)
Benadryl® (diphenhydramine)
Chlor-Trimeton® (chlorpheniramine)

Claritin® (loratadine)
Dimetapp® (contains brompheniramine)
Tavist® (clemastine)
Zyrtec® (cetirizine)

Steroid nasal sprays, listed in the Endocrine (Hormone) System Medications, are also used to control the symptoms of allergy.

Antitussives are used to treat coughs. Examples:

codeine (contained in Robitussin AC® and Phenergan® with codeine)
Delsym® (dextromethorphan)

Hycodan® (hydrocodone/homatropine)
Tessalon® (benzonatate)

Asthma Prophylaxis involves the use of drugs that prevent asthma attacks. Examples:

Accolate® (zafirlukast)
Intal® (cromolyn)
Singulair® (montelukast)
Tilade® (nedocromil)
Zyflo® (zileuton)

Steroid inhalers, listed in the Endocrine (Hormone) System Medications, are also used to prevent asthma attacks.

Bronchodilators relax the airways, so that patients with asthma can breathe more easily. Bronchodilators can be used to stop an asthma attack, as well as prevent them. Examples:

Adrenalin® (epinephrine)
Alupent® (metaproterenol)
Atrovent® (ipratropium)
Brethine® (terbutaline)
Proventil® and Ventolin® (albuterol)
Serevent® (salmeterol)
Theo-Dur® and Elixophyllin® (theophylline)

Decongestants shrink swollen mucus membranes in the nose, so that the nose feels less stuffy. Examples: Neo-Synephrine® (phenylephrine) and Sudafed® (pseudoephedrine). Actifed® is a combination of the antihistamine triprolidine with the decongestant pseudoephedrine.

Expectorants liquefy mucus to help the patient cough up secretions. This will clear a congested chest. Example: Robitussin® (guaifenesin).

Urinary System Medications

Bladder relaxants reduce the muscle spasms of overactive bladder. Examples: Detrol® (tolterodine) and Ditropan® (oxybutynin).

Diuretics decrease excess fluid in the body by increasing the amount of "water" lost through urination. Diuretics are used to lower blood pressure and to treat edema, or swelling. Examples:

Aldactone® (spironolactone)
Demadex® (torsemide)
Dyazide® (triamterene with hydrochlorothiazide)
HydroDiuril® and Oretic® (hydrochlorothiazide)
Lasix® (furosemide)
Lozol® (indapamide)
Zaroxolyn® (metolazone)

Impotence treatments include Viagra® (sildenafil).

Treatments for enlarged prostate, also called Benign Prostatic Hyperplasia (BPH), include:

Flomax® (tamsul<u>osin</u>)　　　　　　Proscar® (finasteride)
Hytrin® (teraz<u>osin</u>)

The bladder relaxants are also used for this purpose.

Chapter Summary

Pharmacies stock hundreds of medications, in a variety of strengths and dosage forms. New drugs are continually joining those already on the pharmacy shelves. A pharmacy clerk should know where new drugs come from, how they are named, and the basic differences between trade name drugs and their generic equivalents. A pharmacy clerk should understand why different dosages are needed and how the various dosage forms are used.

Pharmacists spend years learning pharmacology, so that they can counsel patients and provide detailed drug information. Pharmacy clerks should learn the basics of pharmacology, in order to understand the "language" of pharmacy. Knowing the general pharmacological categories and the common drugs in each will help you understand the importance of your job as a pharmacy clerk and may also help reduce the risk of medication errors.

As you gain experience in the pharmacy, remembering the many drugs and their uses will become easier. If you have questions about a specific medication order, you can always ask your pharmacist. When in doubt about a medication order, always double-check it with the pharmacist—never guess on a customer's order.

Chapter Four • Pharmacology Basics　　　　　　　　　　　　　　　　　　　　　　　　4-35

Name _____

Date _____

Student Enrichment Activities

Fill in the blanks for the following exercises.

1. Explain the difference between the generic, chemical, and trade name of a drug.
   _____
   _____
   _____

2. New drugs are found from the following sources: _____,
   _____, and _____ _____.

3. The trend towards _____ _____ has significantly increased the utilization of generic medications.

4. To be FDA-approved, a new drug must be shown to be _____ and _____.

Complete the following exercises.

5. List at least four oral and four topical dosage forms. _____
   _____
   _____
   _____

6. List the four injectable routes of administration.
   _____
   _____
   _____

Fill in the blanks by looking up the following medications using the appropriate index at the front of the Physician's Desk Reference.

    Generic Name/Trade Name/Product Category

7. Acetaminophen/_____/analgesic, antipyretic

8. acyclovir/Zovirax®/_____

9. _____/Ventolin®/bronchodilator

10. amoxicillin/Amoxil®/_____

11. aspirin/_____/analgesic, antipyretic, anti-inflammatory, NSAID

12. _____/Lotensin®/antihypertensive

13. bumetanide/_____/diuretic

14. cefaclor/Ceclor®/_____

15. cimetidine/Tagamet®/_____

16. _____/Klonopin®/anti-epileptic

17. _____/Valium®/anti-anxiety, anti-epileptic

18. digoxin/Lanoxin®/_____

19. doxycycline/Vibramycin®/_____

Chapter Four • Pharmacology Basics 4-37

Name _____

Date _____

20. erythromycin/_____/antibiotic

21. estrogens/_____/hormones

22. fentanyl/_____/narcotic agonist

23. flurazepam hydrochloride/Dalmane®/_____

24. _____/Lasix®/diuretic

25. _____/Lopid®/antihyperlipidemic

26. guaifenesen/Anti-Tuss®/_____

27. ibuprofen/Advil®/_____

28. insulin/_____/antidiabetic agent

29. _____/Isordil®/anti-anginal agent

30. levothyroxine sodium/Synthroid®/_____

31. lorazepam/_____/anti-anxiety

32. methotrexate/_____/antirheumatic, antineoplastic

33. _____/Lopressor®/antihypertensive

34. _____/MS Contin®/narcotic agonist analgesic

35. naproxen/Naprosyn®/_____

36. _____/Nitro-Bid®/anti-anginal

37. nizatidine/Axid®/_____

38. _____/Cipro®/antibiotic

39. omeprazole/Prilosec®/_____

40. _____/Paxil®/antidepressant

41. _____/Dilantin®/anti-epileptic

42. _____/K-Dur®/electrolyte

43. progesterone/Progestasert®/_____

44. propranolol hydrochloride/_____/beta andrenergic blocker, anti-anginal

45. ranitidine/_____/Histamine 2 blocker

46. sertraline hydrochloride/_____/antidepressant

47. sucralfate/Carafate®/_____

48. tamoxifen citrate/ Nolvadex®/_____

49. temazepam/_____/hypnotic

Chapter Four • Pharmacology Basics 4-39

Name _____

Date _____

50. _____/Theo-Dur®/bronchodilator

51. timolol maleate/Timoptic®/_____

52. trazodone hydrochloride/_____/antidepressant

53. triamcinolone/_____/corticosteroid

54. _____/Coumadin®/anticoagulant

55. _____/Retrovir®/antiviral

Define the following abbreviations.

56. elix: _____

57. gtt: _____

58. AU: _____

59. ung: _____

60. OD: _____

61. Supp: _____

62. sol: _____

63. PO: _____

64. IM: _____

Match the words in Column A with the appropriate description in Column B.

Column A

65. _____ cancer drug

66. _____ lowers blood pressure

67. _____ induces vomiting; treats an overdose

68. _____ decreases blood clotting

69. _____ treats infections caused by viruses

70. _____ slang name for digoxin

71. _____ controls nausea and vomiting

72. _____ stimulates bowel movements

73. _____ treats moderate to severe pain

74. _____ medication placed in the ears

75. _____ reduces anxiety and calms the patient

76. _____ treats bacterial infections

77. _____ insomnia treatment; induces sleep

78. _____ effective in reducing pain, fever, and inflammation

79. _____ drops or ointment used in the eyes

Column B

A. antibiotic
B. anticoagulant
C. anti-emetic
D. antihypertensive
E. antineoplastic
F. antiviral
G. anxiolytic
H. dig
I. emetic
J. hypnotic
K. laxative
L. narcotic analgesic
M. NSAID
N. ophthalmic
O. otic

Chapter Four • Pharmacology Basics

Name _____

Date _____

Match the meaning in Column A with the appropriate term in Column B.

Column A

80. _____ an unintended reaction

81. _____ the desired response to a drug

82. _____ an unpredictable reaction to a drug caused by genetics or other factors specific to that person

83. _____ an effect that blocks or works against an action

84. _____ an excessive sensitivity to a chemical substance, causing rash or difficulty breathing

85. _____ resistance to a drug, such that increased doses are needed to produce the desired therapeutic effect

86. _____ an unfavorable effect or toxicity in response to a drug

87. _____ an excessive response to the usual dose of a drug, causing exaggerated effects

88. _____ the combined effects of two or more agents acting together

89. _____ to use more or less of a substance to achieve a desired result

Column B

A. synergistic effect

B. antagonistic effect

C. side effect

D. adverse drug reaction

E. therapeutic effect

F. idiosyncratic reaction

G. allergic reaction

H. tolerance

I. sensitivity

J. titrate

Chapter Five
The Prescription

Objectives

After completing this chapter, you should be able to do the following:

1. Define and correctly spell each of the key terms.

2. Accurately use the most common abbreviations used in the pharmacy.

3. Define the standard units of measurement used in the pharmacy.

4. Describe a properly filled out prescription blank.

5. Describe the importance of patient confidentiality.

6. Describe several examples of warning/auxiliary labels.

7. Discuss methods of spotting fraudulent prescriptions.

8. Describe what to do if there is a theft in the pharmacy.

Key Terms

- apothecary and avoirdupois systems
- confidential
- fraudulent
- interdependence
- metric system
- reimbursable
- strength
- warning/auxiliary labels

Introduction

When a customer leaves a pharmacy with medication, a team of professionals has completed a process that began with a prescriber filling out a prescription blank. Many times, the customer is not aware of the number of people who have contributed to the filling of the prescription. The team shares an **interdependence**. The patients and customers see the results of the team effort.

interdependence: actions or activities that require one person to work with another.

Working with prescriptions means dealing with systems of numbers, symbols, and abbreviations. These systems are designed to simplify prescription processing, although they can lead to misinterpretation and error. It is critically important that the numbers, symbols, and abbreviations be learned correctly. However, when in doubt, clarification must be made.

This chapter will introduce the various systems used to provide information on prescriptions. This chapter will also describe the processing of prescriptions.

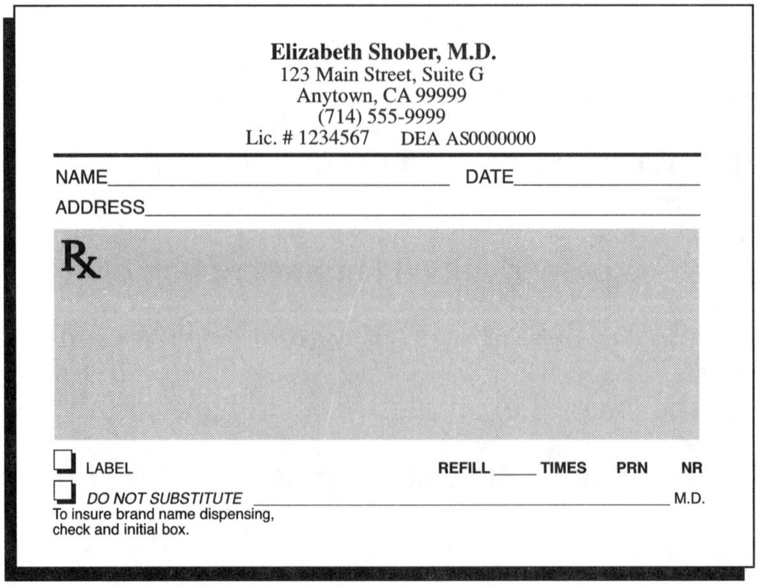
Elizabeth Shober, M.D.
123 Main Street, Suite G
Anytown, CA 99999
(714) 555-9999
Lic. # 1234567 DEA AS0000000

NAME______________ DATE__________
ADDRESS______________

℞

☐ LABEL REFILL____ TIMES PRN NR
☐ *DO NOT SUBSTITUTE* ______________ M.D.
To insure brand name dispensing, check and initial box.

Figure 5-1: A Prescription Blank

The Elements of a Prescription

A prescription is an order from a prescriber for a medication or treatment for a specific patient. Most prescriptions are handwritten by a physician. Review Chapter Two for information on other classifications of prescribers and other methods of prescription transmission to the pharmacy.

A prescription is a legal document. In addition to identifying the patient by name and address, a prescription has four main parts:

- *Superscription:* represented by the "Rx" symbol, which means "Take."
- *Inscription:* the name of the drug (trade or generic) and the **strength** of medication being prescribed. Occasionally a prescription will be written for a compounded formula. In that case, the inscription contains the names of the ingredients and their quantities.
- *Subscription:* the directions to the pharmacist or technician filling the prescription. This includes the dosage form (tablet, capsule, syrup, etc.) and the total amount of drug to be dispensed.
- *Signatura:* Often called the "sig." This provides the directions for use that patient must follow, including how large each dose will be and how often to take the medication. Special instructions, such as "with meals," or "as needed for pain" may be part of the sig. The "sig" must be accurately translated into terms the patient can understand and follow before it is placed on the label.

> **strength:** the amount of drug contained in each tablet, capsule, or teaspoonful of a medication. For liquids, this is sometimes called the *concentration*.

The prescription may also contain the number of refills authorized by the prescriber and information on using generic substitutes.

The prescriber's name, license classification (MD, DDS, etc.), address, and telephone number appear on preprinted prescription forms. Prescriptions for controlled substances must also show the prescriber's **DEA** number. To complete the prescription, the prescriber must sign it.

Prescription Processing – Part 1

When a customer comes in to get a prescription filled, be sure the prescription information is complete. Often the patient's address and/or telephone number is missing. It is essential to get this information before submitting the prescription to be filled. Also, check the spelling of the patient's name. If it is a common name, such as Jones or Smith, be sure to get the customer's middle initial. This will help avoid mixing prescription bottles when names are similar. Also obtain the patient's birth date. This assists the pharmacist in determining the age of the patient.

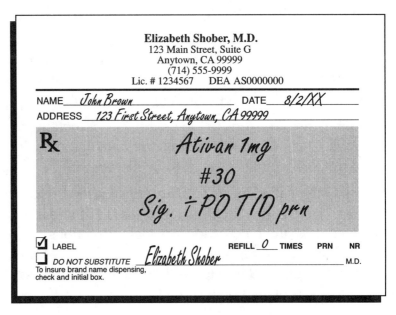

Figure 5-2: A Properly Filled Out Prescription

At this time, ask customers if they will be paying for the prescription with cash, a check, a credit card, an insurance card, or state funded reimbursement. This information is very important, as each plan has specific medications that are **reimbursable** and those that are not. Most insurance plans specify that a generic drug should be substituted for the brand name drug when available. Get as much information as possible so future problems and delays are avoided. Obtain copies of cards (front and back) or other identification before the customer leaves the counter.

If a customer does not have the necessary information, offer the use of the telephone to aid the customer in obtaining the information. Check your facility's policy on supplying medication when no insurance information is available. For pharmacy clerks working in retail pharmacies, additional customer infor-

reimbursable: in a pharmacy, medications for which the patient's insurance company has agreed to provide payment.

mation can be obtained from the physician prescribing the medication. Calling the prescriber's office staff generally results in getting all necessary information to process the prescription.

Always let the customer know if the medication is listed in the formulary used by his or her insurance company, if they are expecting the cost of the drug to be covered this way. Not all medications ordered are covered by all insurance companies. Many insurance companies require a co-pay. Be sure to let the customer know how much this costs.

Once the information has been verified, place the prescription in the area designated for filling. Each facility will have its own system for completing orders. Make sure prescriptions are placed in the order in which the customers arrive. People are very aware of who arrived first when they are waiting for service—especially in pharmacies. Many pharmacy customers have already waited in doctor's offices or clinics to be seen, and they may not be as understanding as they would be in normal circumstances. Explain delays if they occur. People respond better when they are informed about the situation.

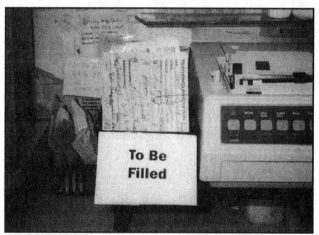

Figure 5-3: Place prescriptions to be filled in the appropriate location.

In some areas, the pharmacy clerk participates in prescription processing by inputting the prescription information into the pharmacy computer. The computer then produces the label that will be placed on the patient's medication and the other records that document the dispensing process, including the receipt for the prescription. Many pharmacy computers will automatically bill third-party payors for prescriptions by using on-line claims processing. Therefore, the information entered into the computer must be exact. If it isn't exact, the label, receipt, prescription records, and billing all will be incorrect.

To accurately input prescription data, the pharmacy clerk must know the abbreviations and measurement systems used in pharmacy. Common prescription abbreviations and measurements appear in the following two sections.

Abbreviations

Healthcare workers use abbreviations to increase the speed and efficiency of their communications. Most medication orders contain numerous abbreviations, indicating the amount of medication to use, the route of administration, and the dosing interval. Some drugs, such as aspirin (ASA) and nitroglycerin (NTG), are even ordered by their abbreviated names.

Although abbreviations allow the pharmacy staff to work faster and easier, they can also lead to mistakes, which might harm the patient. Accuracy in writing and interpreting abbreviations is critical to patient safety. Poor penmanship can lead to errors in interpretation of abbreviations. Since some abbreviations have more than one meaning, it is important to look at each abbreviation in its context. If there is any doubt as to the meaning of an abbreviation, it must be clarified.

In addition to the lists of commonly used abbreviations shown in this chapter, each hospital has its own list of accepted abbreviations. The Joint Commission on Accreditation of Health Care Organizations requires this list to be kept in a policy manual that is available for all employees. Abbreviations not found on the list are not considered appropriate for use. Be sure all abbreviations meet the hospital's standards.

Figures 5-4 through 5-8 include common abbreviations used in the pharmacy. Many of these abbreviations can be written in either upper or lower case letters, without changing their meanings. Practice in writing and using abbreviations is necessary to become proficient in their use. Remember: When in doubt, ASK!

Chapter Five • The Prescription

5-7

Abbreviations: Dosing Intervals

ā	before	PRN	as needed
ac	before meals	q̄	every
ad lib	as desired	qAM	every morning
AM	morning	QD	every day
ASAP	as soon as possible	q4h	every four hours
BID	twice a day	QID	four times a day
c̄	with	QOD	every other day
d	day	qPM	every evening
h	hour	rep	repeat
hs	bedtime (hour of sleep)	STAT	NOW!, immediately
mo	month	TID	three times a day
p̄	after	UD	as directed
pc	after meals	wk	week
PM	evening		

Figure 5-4: Abbreviations for the Frequency of Medication Administration

Measurements Used in the Pharmacy

There are several measurement systems used in the pharmacy today. The "common systems" (apothecary and avoirdupois) are used occasionally, although the metric system is becoming the standard for medication orders. On the other hand, patients will most often measure their doses in household units. Converting between the systems of measurement is sometimes necessary when preparing prescription labels.

The **apothecary** and **avoirdupois systems** measure weights and volumes in units that have been used for centuries. Although these common systems are being replaced by the metric system, it is important to recognize the remaining common units of measure. The grain (gr) is occasionally used to indicate the strength of medications such as codeine and thyroid. Very rarely, a prescriber will use the minim symbol (♏) to indicate a measurement in *drops*.

Other common system measurements that are still in use are shared with the household system. You may be familiar with these because they are often used for grocery products. These common system measurements include ounces (oz), pints (pt), quarts (qt), gallons (gal), and pounds (lb).

apothecary and **avoirdupois systems:** rarely used systems of weights and measures that use specific ratios of grains, ounces, minims, quarts, and pounds.

Sometimes confusion exists with the apothecary measurement of the fluid dram (f ʒ). When written on a prescription or medication order, *f ʒ* means that the medication is to be measured in *teaspoonfuls* (tsp). As with all apothecary measurements, the number of teaspoonfuls is indicated by a lower case Roman numeral listed after the f ʒ symbol. For example, *f ʒ ii* means that a patient is to take *two teaspoonfuls* of drug. Sometimes, to indicate that they are lower case, Roman numerals may have a line along the top of the number, as follows: ī.

Another apothecary measurement is used as a symbol for one tablespoonful (tbsp). Although it technically means one-half fluid ounce, *f ʒ ss* should be translated as *one tablespoonful* when put on a prescription label.

Fluid ounces are also used to measure the volume of medication to be dispensed on a prescription. For example, *f ℥ iv* means that *four fluid ounces* of the medication should be poured into the prescription bottle. If a medication is clearly a liquid, the prescriber may leave off the "f" in either the fluid dram or fluid ounce symbols.

Abbreviations: Roman Numerals

i, ī	1	xii, x̄iī	12
ii, īi	2	xv, x̄v̄	15
iii, īiī	3	xvi, x̄vī	16
iv, īv̄	4	xx, x̄x̄	20
v, v̄	5	xxx, x̄x̄x̄	30
vi, v̄ī	6	L	50
vii, v̄iī	7	C	100
viii, v̄iiī	8	D	500
ix, īx̄	9	M	1,000
x, x̄	10	ss	½

Figure 5-5: Roman Numeral Abbreviations

metric system: a uniform system of measurement that uses the meter, gram, and liter as the units of measurement, based on units of ten.

The **metric system** is the most used measuring system throughout the world. The basic units of the metric system are the liter (L), a volume measurement, and the gram (g), a weight measurement. Some healthcare providers continue to use "Gm" as the symbol for gram, although "g" is the official abbreviation. As with other abbreviations, a capital letter may be used, rather than the lower case. The basic unit of length in the metric system is the meter (m). However, measurements of length are rarely used in pharmacy.

In healthcare, the most frequently used metric measurements are all multiples of 1000 of the basic units. The Latin prefix *milli-* means one-thousandth. Therefore, a *milliliter (mL)* is one-thousandth of a liter. A cubic centimeter (cc) is identical to a milliliter. 1 cc = 1 mL. One liter could be written as either 1000 mL or 1000 cc.

$$1 L = 1,000 mL = 1,000 cc$$

A *milligram (mg)* is one-thousandth of a gram. Measurements of weight can be made even smaller by using the prefix *micro-*. A *microgram (mcg)* is one-thousandth of a milligram, or one-millionth of a gram.

$$1 g = 1,000 mg$$

$$1 mg = 1,000 mcg$$

$$1 g = 1,000,000 mcg$$

When expressing a patient's weight in the metric system, the unit *kilogram* is used. A kilogram is a much larger weight, equivalent to 1000 grams.

$$1 kg = 1,000 g$$

Converting between the metric and common systems can be particularly confusing, because there isn't agreement as to what some of the equivalents really are. Figure 5-6 presents the *approximate* equivalents used in prescription ordering and dispensing. These equivalents are different from the exact conversions used in the manufacturing and commercial packaging of medications.

For example, a fluid ounce is usually ordered and dispensed as *30 milliliters*. An ounce of a cream or ointment is often ordered and dispensed as *30 grams*. These "dispensing ounces" are larger than the exact metric equivalents that the manufacturers use. Manufacturers package 29.57 milliliters per fluidounce, which means they will put 473 milliliters in a pint, instead of 480 milliliters. A one-ounce tube may contain only 28.35 grams of cream or ointment, not the 30 grams that you might expect. Manufacturers can save money by packaging their products using the smaller, exact equivalents.

Approximate Measurement Equivalents

Weight

METRIC		COMMON
60 milligrams (mg)	=	1 grain (gr)
30 grams (g)	=	1 ounce (oz)
454 grams (g)	=	1 pound (lb) = 16 ounces

Volume

METRIC		COMMON
5 milliliters (mL)	=	1 teaspoonful (f ʒ)
15 milliliters (mL)	=	1 tablespoonful (f ʒ ss)
30 milliliters (mL)	=	1 fluid ounce (oz) = f ʒ i
473 milliliters (mL)	=	1 pint (pt) = 16 fluid ounces
946 milliliters (mL)	=	1 quart (qt) = 32 fluid ounces
3785 milliliters (mL)	=	1 gallon (gal) = 128 fluid ounces

Figure 5-6: Approximate Metric Equivalents Chart

Abbreviations: Measurements

cc	cubic centimeter	**mL**	milliliter
g, G, Gm	gram	**no.**	number
gal	gallon	**oz, ʒ**	ounce
gr	grain	**f ʒ**	fluid ounce
L	liter	**pt**	pint
lb	pound	**qt**	quart
mEq	milliEquivalent	**f ʒ, tsp**	teaspoon, dram
mcg	microgram	**f ʒ ss, tbsp**	one tablespoon
mg	milligram		

Figure 5-7: Measurement Abbreviations

Chapter Five • The Prescription

Abbreviations: Miscellaneous

BP	blood pressure	**s̄**	without
c̄	with	**Sig**	directions for the patient
D/C	discontinue	**sx**	symptoms
Disp	dispense	**T, temp**	temperature
HA	headache	**<**	less than
non rep	no refill	**>**	more than
N/V	nausea and vomiting	**↑**	increase
qs, qsad	fill up to	**↓**	decrease
Rx	prescription; take		

Figure 5-8: Miscellaneous Abbreviations

Prescription Labels

Each pharmacy will have a standard format for its prescription labels, taking into consideration the requirements of state and federal law. The computer will produce labels to follow that format. Although the positioning of information may be different, there are similarities in prescription labels. Each label will probably include the following information:

- The pharmacy's name, address, and telephone number.

- The prescription number: a unique number that identifies this prescription and allows pharmacy personnel to retrieve the documents related to the prescription.

- Directions for use, spelled out clearly and completely in terms the patient can understand.

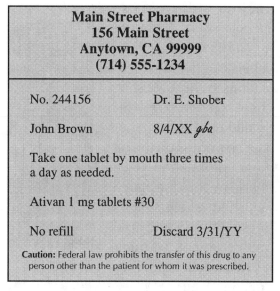

Figure 5-9: A Sample Prescription Label

- The dispensing date: the date the prescription was filled or refilled. This may be different than the date the prescription was written. Some labels will also include the original prescription date on labels for refills.
- The prescriber's name and perhaps his or her license classification.
- The patient's full name.
- The medication name, strength, dosage form, quantity, and manufacturer (if generic).
- Refill information: the number of refills remaining, or a time limit on refills, or both.
- The **beyond-use** or **expiration date**: the date after which the medication should be thrown out, if the patient has not finished all of it.
- The initials of the pharmacist responsible for dispensing the prescription. State law may require that the pharmacist hand initial any label generated by a pharmacy clerk or technician.

Warning/Auxiliary Labels

Patient-oriented practice means that the pharmacist and his or her staff work to prevent complications from medication use. Many medications have side effects that are potentially hazardous to the patient. Some of these effects include drowsiness, sleeplessness, **agitation**, or nausea. Auxiliary labels are affixed to medications to alert the user to these potential problems. In addition, many labels can be printed on the patient information sheet that is given to the patient with the receipt for the prescription. Some of the most common **warning/auxiliary labels** are illustrated in Figure 5-11.

warning/auxiliary labels: additional labels attached to a patient's prescription bottle, giving directions regarding the use or storage of the medication, or announcing potentially harmful effects of the medication.

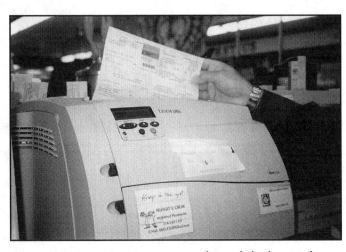

Figure 5-10: Warning or auxiliary labels can be affixed to the prescription bottle or printed on the patient information sheet.

Chapter Five • The Prescription

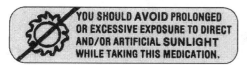
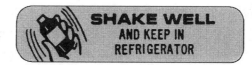
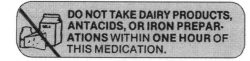
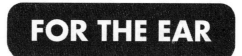
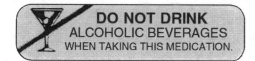

Figure 5-11: Common Warning/Auxiliary Labels

Prescription Processing – Part 2

The pharmacist or technician will complete the prescription dispensing process by selecting the correct medication, counting it, and putting it into a proper container. If the technician has filled the prescription, the pharmacist will verify that it was done correctly. Once the prescription is filled, it is placed in the area designated for completed prescriptions.

When the prescription is ready, call the customer by name to pick it up. This ensures that the correct person gets the correct medication. Repeat customers' names when they come to the counter, especially if several people are waiting for prescriptions. If there is any doubt about the customer's identity, ask to see a driver's license or other picture ID. Remember that the person picking up the prescription may not be the patient; it may be a relative or family friend.

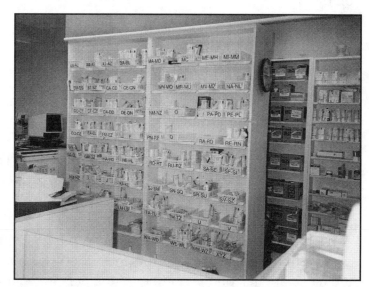

Figure 5-12: An Area Designated for Completed Prescriptions

When the customer pays for the medication, include the receipt in the bag with the medication. There may be a computerized receipt and a standard cash register receipt. The patient may need both for his or her financial records. Include any other paperwork, such as printed patient information sheets.

Many states require that a pharmacist counsel patients on the proper use of each new prescription medication. Some states also require counseling on prescription refills. Even if counseling is not required, it is important to ask all customers if they have questions about their medications. Many pharmacies have consultation areas where the pharmacist and patient can speak with each other privately. Escort patients with questions to the consultation area and let the pharmacist know that the patient is waiting. If a patient is reluctant to talk with the pharmacist in person, point out the pharmacy's telephone number on the prescription label. Patients can call from home if they have questions or problems.

confidential: private; not to be discussed with others.

Remember that prescription labels contain **confidential** information. Do not leave prescription bottles on the counter or allow other customers to read the labels. It is best to put the prescription bottles into a bag as soon as they are taken off the shelf.

Taking Telephone Orders

When a prescriber's office calls to order a new prescription, transfer the call to the pharmacist immediately. Only a pharmacist may take a new prescription order. Before placing the call on hold, get the caller's name, phone number, and the name of the patient. This will assist the pharmacist taking the call. It will also allow the pharmacist to call back if the prescriber's office is accidentally disconnected.

A patient or the patient's representative may call in to request a refill on a prescription. Be sure to ask for the prescription number, the patient's name, and the name and telephone number of the person making the call. It is helpful to find out if there are refills allowed on the prescription. Put the caller on hold while you check. If there are no refills allowed, let the caller know that the refill will have to be authorized by the prescriber. Getting refill authorization can take several hours to a day or more. For that reason, many pharmacies encourage patients to call at least 24 hours before they plan to pick up their refill medication.

Keep in mind that there are restrictions on certain refills, even if the prescription shows that refills remain. Since abuse can be an issue, pharmacists calculate the time between refills on controlled substances. Third-party payors also limit refills based on the number of days supply of drug that has been dispensed. If there are any questions about whether the patient can have a medication refilled, ask the pharmacist.

When taking a telephone request for a refill, ask the caller when the medication will be picked up. If a medication has to be special ordered for the patient, or if refill authorization has to be obtained, the refill may not be ready when the patient plans to pick it up. It is much better to find that out before the patient makes a trip to the pharmacy.

Patient Confidentiality

Pharmacy records contain a great deal of information about a patient's medical conditions and the drugs taken to treat those conditions. Because all patients have a right to privacy, their medical information must be kept confidential. Legally and ethically, confidentiality must be observed by all healthcare workers.

While it may be tempting to talk about patients outside of the pharmacy, this would breach the patients' confidentiality. Even within the pharmacy, discussion about a patient's medications or condition should be done only with those who have a need to know.

Breaching a patient's confidentiality is sometimes done unintentionally. Be aware that customers may be able to hear what is said behind the pharmacy counter, even if it doesn't appear that they're listening. Also be cautious about telephone requests for information about prescriptions that have been filled in the pharmacy. Some pharmacies wait to provide such information until they have been able to verify that the caller has a legal right to the information. Insurance companies are aware of the patient's right to confidentiality and are usually willing to wait for the information.

Proper disposal of pharmacy paperwork is also a key to maintaining confidentiality. Pharmacies have become very aware of the need to destroy written documents that identify patients and their medications. Outdated prescriptions may be shredded in the pharmacy or might be sent to a company that specializes in destroying sensitive records. Some pharmacies even shred the notes taken when patients call in their refill requests, after the refills have been processed.

Confidentiality is an absolute right. Breaching a patient's confidentiality puts a pharmacy employee at risk of being terminated and could put the pharmacy at risk of a lawsuit. Respect the patient's right to privacy.

In Real Life . . .

> Taniqua is working as a pharmacy clerk at Maple Street Drug Store. One afternoon, Leonard and Mai Lin come in to pick up some OTC cough syrup for their son. Taniqua finishes ringing up a prescription for Mrs. Garcia and then goes out to help Leonard and Mai Lin find the product they are looking for.
>
> Taniqua has been friends with Leonard and Mai Lin since high school, so they chat for a moment about old times. Then Leonard mentions that he noticed Taniqua waiting on Mrs. Garcia, who happens to be a neighbor of Leonard's mom. Leonard tells Taniqua that the neighborhood has been concerned about Mrs. Garcia lately. She just doesn't seem to be herself. Maybe Taniqua knows what's wrong? If Taniqua could just give them a little information, Leonard could tell his mom – and then she might be able to help Mrs. Garcia.
>
> Taniqua knows what's wrong with Mrs. Garcia. She's been coming in to the pharmacy nearly every week for the past month to pick up her medications. Taniqua knows that Mrs. Garcia is taking an antidepressant and a medication to control anxiety. Taniqua also knows that these medications, as well as the conditions they're treating, could cause Mrs. Garcia to act differently.

Chapter Five • The Prescription

Discussion Questions

1. What should Taniqua say to Leonard? How much information should she share?

2. Taniqua is friends with Leonard and Mai Lin. Does this make a difference in the situation?

3. Leonard just wants to help Mrs. Garcia. How does this affect her right to privacy?

4. If you were in Mrs. Garcia's position, what would you want Taniqua to do?

Fraudulent Prescriptions

Obtaining medication fraudulently is a federal crime. Despite this, you may come across fraud while working in the pharmacy. The pharmacy clerk should be alert to any signs that a prescription is not authentic. Some warning signs are listed below.

- The number of refills or the number to be dispensed looks like it may have been altered. (Roman numerals are especially easy to alter.)
- The prescription is from an out of town prescriber who cannot be reached by telephone.
- The DEA number is missing.
- A physician comes in with a script for a patient and says he or she will deliver it.

It is the pharmacist's ultimate responsibility to spot a **fraudulent** prescription. However, it is everyone's job to be alert to suspicious people. If you suspect a prescription is fraudulent, it is important NOT to confront the person yourself. Each facility will have its own policy for handling situations like this. Ask the pharmacist for information on how to handle this situation.

fraudulent: unauthorized, false, forged.

Pharmacy Theft

One of the most serious issues confronting all retail sales businesses is the potential for robbery and theft. This is especially true of pharmacies in large urban centers. Pharmacies throughout the country are developing ways to minimize the risk to employees who may be victims in a robbery.

There are a few basic rules to follow. It is important for you to discuss this subject as soon as you begin work. The entire pharmacy team must be aware of the facility's policy on how to respond to a robber's threats. The most basic rule is DO NOT RESIST!

Police authorities believe that robbery victims should not confront the criminal in any way during a crime. Following the robber's instructions greatly increases the chance of survival for all employees. Do not make any sudden movements or attempt to communicate in code with other employees.

To prevent shoplifting, be aware of who is coming in and going out of the pharmacy. Do not spend prolonged periods of time in back supply rooms or in areas where you can't see the customers. Watch people who are shopping in the pharmacy or who are browsing as they wait for their prescriptions. Be suspicious of people who seem to be loitering without purpose.

Far more common than robberies or shoplifting are employee thefts. In fact, employee theft presents the most serious source of loss to businesses. The pharmacy is a unique place to work. Many specialized medications and products are readily available to staff members. Some have found the temptation too great to resist. Be aware that since 1984, it is a federal crime to steal more than $500 worth of narcotics. Most people do not realize the seriousness of taking drugs that are not prescribed for them. In addition to committing a federal crime, the loss of trust will most likely result in dismissal. Pharmacies rely on the honesty of their employees more than most businesses. Stealing medication, especially narcotics, jeopardizes the entire pharmacy, not just the person who is stealing.

Thieves may want to befriend pharmacy employees for the sole purpose of obtaining drugs. Be alert for people who suddenly take an interest in where you work. Be especially concerned if the person has a drug abuse history. These people may begin to pressure you to steal medication to support their drug habit. Let the proper authorities know if you are being approached by such people.

If you know another employee is taking drugs, it is your legal responsibility to report it. In addition to saving your job, you may also help the person to begin a recovery program. Many times, the person enters a **rehabilitation** program as a result of being caught.

Chapter Summary

Working in a pharmacy means decoding information written in abbreviations and symbols. Pharmacy clerks can use their knowledge of prescription format, abbreviations, and symbols to speed up prescription processing, by ensuring that information appears complete. Pharmacy clerks who enter prescription data into the computer must be very skilled in reading prescriptions accurately. Although the pharmacist has the ultimate responsibility for the accuracy of the prescriptions dispensed, all pharmacy personnel can help prevent medication errors.

Occasionally, theft occurs in pharmacies. Whether it is through a fraudulent prescription, shoplifting, or robbery, pharmacy clerks must be concerned for their personal safety and the safety of their coworkers. When a fellow employee is the thief, other staff members must be courageous enough to report the theft.

Chapter Five • The Prescription

Name _____
Date _____

Student Enrichment Activities

Complete the following exercises.

1. Describe the essential patient information needed before submitting a prescription to be filled.

   _____
   _____
   _____

2. List the information included in each of the following components of a prescription.
   superscription: _____
   inscription: _____
   subscription: _____
   signatura: _____

3. List five examples of warning/auxiliary labels.
   A. _____
   B. _____
   C. _____
   D. _____
   E. _____

4. Patient confidentiality is important because: _____
   _____
   _____
   _____
   _____

5-21

5. List four signs that a prescription might be fraudulent.

   A. _____

   B. _____

   C. _____

   D. _____

Circle T for True, or F for False.

6. T F Auxiliary/warning labels are used to alert the patient to important information and potential problems related to the medication being taken.

7. T F The apothecary system is the most widely used measurement system in the world.

8. T F In most pharmacies, employee theft accounts for more financial loss than shoplifting or robberies.

9. T F One fluid ounce is the same as 1000 cc.

10. T F Fraudulent prescriptions may be identified by alterations in the number of refills allowed or changes to the quantity ordered.

11. T F Do not resist if you are being robbed in a pharmacy.

Chapter Five • The Prescription   5-23

Name _____
Date _____

Write out each of the following Sigs in complete sentences.

12. Tabs iii po q4h prn HA
    _____

13. ʒ ss PO TID
    _____

14. Caps ii po q6h
    _____

15. ʒ i po BID (AM & HS)
    _____

16. Supp i PR q6h prn constipation
    _____

17. Gtts ii AS q3-4h
    _____

18. Tab i PO TID ac
    _____

19. Gtts ii OU qid PRN
    _____

20. Supp ss PR q6-8h prn T> 101
    _____

21. Apply to rash QID UD
    _____

22. Tabs s̄s̄ po qod
   _____

23. Gtt i-ii AU prn pain
   _____

24. Caps ii po qHS x 2 wk
   _____

25. Supp i PR q8h prn N/V
   _____

26. Tab i po qAM for BP control
   _____

27. Caps ii BID prn cough
   _____

28. ʒ ī TID pc
   _____

29. Gtts ii OD q10-12h
   _____

30. Tabs īs̄s̄ po q4h prn cold sx
   _____

31. Caps iv stat, ii BID x 10d
   _____

Chapter Six
Inventory Control in the Pharmacy

Objectives

After completing this chapter, you should be able to do the following:

1. Define and correctly spell each of the key terms.

2. Explain the difference between stocking shelves in the retail and the hospital pharmacy.

3. Discuss how filling patient medication orders is accomplished in both a retail and a hospital pharmacy.

4. Discuss the responsibilities involved in transporting medications within the hospital and to customers' homes.

5. Explain the importance of recording patient medication use.

6. Discuss how medications and supplies are billed and reordered.

Key Terms

- aseptic technique
- back-ordered
- chart orders
- expiration date
- IV piggyback
- multi-dose vial
- NDC number
- perpetual inventory
- pharmacy patient profile
- shelf life
- sundries
- unit dose
- vendor

Introduction

Maintaining, managing, and accounting for inventory is one of the most important functions of the pharmacy clerk. Keeping adequate supplies of medications and medical equipment is critical to maintaining good customer service. Pharmacy clerks will find that a large portion of their job includes stocking shelves and ordering supplies. The importance of these duties cannot be overstated.

Inventory control involves maintaining an adequate stock of medications, as well as storing those medications in a safe and secure manner. It also means keeping track of the purchasing and distribution of medications. Good inventory control allows the pharmacy to have enough medications on hand to fill prescriptions and orders, without having so much stock that drugs deteriorate before they can be used.

shelf life: the length of time a product can be kept in stock before its contents are altered by age.

expiration date: the date after which the stability and potency of a drug cannot be guaranteed; also called the beyond-use date.

Shelf Life

Each drug has a **shelf life** based on its stability. The manufacturer indicates the shelf life for each drug by assigning it an **expiration date** or beyond-use date. After the expiration date, the potency of the drug can no longer be guaranteed. Medications should never be sold beyond their expiration date. The pharmacy staff must take care to routinely check the expiration dates of both the prescription and OTC products kept in stock. Expired products must be removed from stock and disposed of according to the pharmacy's policy.

Chapter Six • Inventory Control in the Pharmacy

Patients should also be alerted to the importance of the expiration date on their prescription medications. Although it is not safe to do so, many people keep bottles of old medications at home—well past the labeled expiration date. After the expiration date, most medications are no longer at full strength; that means that they won't be as effective. Some medications, however, can become toxic and dangerous for the patients to take after the expiration date.

It is possible for a drug to lose its potency before the expiration date. This occurs if the drug is stored in improper conditions. To improve stability, some drugs must be stored in the refrigerator or freezer. Many drugs must be protected from light and excess humidity. Always read the labels on drug bottles to ensure that the correct storage conditions are being maintained. Keep medication lids tightly closed to prevent moisture from damaging the drugs.

Purchasing

Each pharmacy will purchase medications from a number of different **vendors**. Buying medications "direct" means that the drugs are purchased directly from their manufacturers. Pharmacies usually buy a few drug products direct, though most are purchased through a wholesaler. A wholesaler acts like a supermarket for drugs, carrying products from many different companies. Wholesalers often carry OTC items, pharmacy supplies, and **sundries**, as well as prescription medications.

It is important to know which drug products are purchased from which vendors. In many cases, the pharmacy will have a contract to buy certain medications from a "prime vendor." The contract guarantees a lower price for the pharmacy and it may entitle the pharmacy to special services from the vendor. If a medication is **back-ordered** from the prime vendor, then secondary vendors will be used.

Many vendors are now using on-line or electronic transmission systems for drug purchasing. These systems are much faster and more accurate than the telephone ordering that was common in the past. These systems use either a bar code or a numeric identifier for each drug product, which reduces the risk of ordering an incorrect product. Since each bar code or number is unique, there is no confusion as to which drug product is being ordered. Some vendors assign their own six or seven digit number to each product they carry. Others use the manufacturer's **NDC number** for the drugs.

> **vendor:** a company that sells a drug. This may be the manufacturer or a wholesaler.
>
> **sundries:** various small items often sold in a pharmacy, such as safety pins, bandages, sunglasses, etc.
>
> **back-ordered:** temporarily unavailable from the supplier. Also referred to as "short."
>
> **NDC number:** a unique number that identifies each drug product. The NDC number indicates the name of the manufacturer and the name, strength, dosage form, and package size of the drug product.

Another advantage of on-line and electronically transmitted orders is that the pharmacy will know immediately if a drug is back-ordered, or "short." When a patient is waiting for a medication to arrive, it is important to know if a vendor cannot supply the product quickly. This information allows the pharmacy to try to purchase the drug from a different vendor without undue delay.

In large hospitals, health systems, or chain drug stores, purchasing may be done through a purchasing agent or buyer. These large groups may act as their own wholesalers, keeping drug products in a central warehouse for distribution to individual pharmacies as needed. The pharmacy staff then requisitions the drugs through the buyer, rather than from the individual vendors.

Most pharmacies purchase on a daily basis, so that "fast-movers" can be restocked. Some wholesalers are able to give same-day delivery for medication orders placed before noon. Fast delivery is one advantage of buying from the wholesalers, which usually are local companies. Buying direct may mean ordering from a company in another state, which can delay delivery for several days.

Keeping track of the inventory is also a part of inventory control. Many pharmacies decide what to order using an "eyeball inventory" system. During the day, staff members keep track of medications that are being sold by writing them down in a "want book" or by punching the numeric identifiers into an electronic or on-line ordering device. At the end of the day, the orders are transmitted to the vendors.

Bar codes have simplified the ordering process. As drugs are used to fill prescriptions or sold OTC, the bar codes on the containers are scanned. Bar code systems are able to keep a **perpetual inventory** of drugs that have been used, automatically creating an order for replacements.

perpetual inventory: an on-going system of tracking drugs received in the pharmacy and sold by the pharmacy.

Controlled Substances

Pharmacies are required to keep detailed records of the purchase and use of Schedule II drugs. Because Schedule II drugs include the narcotics and other drugs with high abuse potential, the pharmacist will closely monitor this type of drug stock. Schedule II drugs must be ordered on special order forms provided by the government. They are delivered in separate orders, which must be signed for by the pharmacist. The law requires each pharmacy to do a physical count of the Schedule II drugs, at least every two years. This involves counting *every tablet and capsule* of all Schedule II drugs and recording those numbers in an inventory record.

Stocking Shelves

The pharmacy clerk may spend a lot of time stocking the shelves in the pharmacy. It is important to learn the basic arrangement of the pharmacy inventory so that stock can be put away quickly and accurately.

Pharmacy stock must be kept under the proper storage conditions, including refrigeration or freezing, if indicated by the manufacturer. When stocking drugs, make sure to read the product labels and look for special storage requirements. If a drug that needs refrigeration is put on a regular shelf, it may quickly deteriorate and have to be discarded. Drug products are very expensive, so this could be a major dollar loss to the pharmacy.

Pharmacies are required to store oral medications separately from the topicals. (Review Chapter Four for the types of dosage forms in each group.) The pharmacy will also keep specific dosage forms together, such as the ophthalmics or the inhalers. This allows the pharmacist or the technician to quickly locate the medication needed to fill a specific prescription.

Controlled substances are usually stored in locked drawers or cabinets. Large pharmacies may have a locked narcotic vault or room, depending on the amount of controlled substances stock the pharmacy has. Access to the narcotic storage area is usually restricted to the pharmacist or a specially trained technician.

The antineoplastics, or cancer chemotherapy drugs, are often stored in a segregated location within the pharmacy. These drugs are highly toxic. Extra caution must be taken in storing and handling these drugs. They must be prevented from spilling or splashing, because of the potential damage they can cause.

Within each group, medications will be arranged alphabetically. Some pharmacies alphabetize using the trade names of the drugs, while others use the generic names. This can cause confusion until the pharmacy clerk becomes more familiar with the drug names. Chapter Four lists both the trade and generic names of most of the Top 200 prescription drugs. The *American Drug Index* (also discussed in Chapter Four) is a good reference to use to quickly look up the trade or generic name of a drug that you are not familiar with. When in doubt, though, ask the pharmacist.

Stocking Shelves in a Retail Pharmacy

Retail customers often come into the pharmacy to purchase more than just their prescription medications. Therefore, there is considerable space designated for over-the-counter (OTC) medications, equipment, health and beauty aids, and sundries in even the smallest pharmacy. These shelves must be neat and pleasing to the customer's eye. Many pharmacies will designate specific shelf space for certain products. This is done to enhance sales of high demand and potentially high profit products, as well as for the customers' convenience.

In retail pharmacies, it is particularly important to keep the shelves stocked in the OTC sales area. If a particular item is out of stock, you will probably receive directions to supply the area with other products. Empty shelves can create a negative impression to customers. Retailers would rather have an item overstocked on a shelf than leave a space empty.

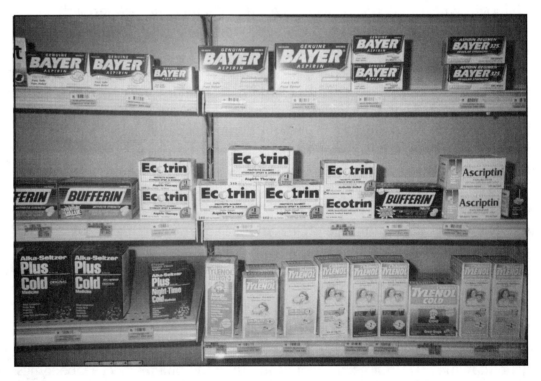

Figure 6-1: Over-the-counter (OTC) medications are also sold in many retail pharmacies.

Chapter Six • Inventory Control in the Pharmacy

In addition to the retail merchandise, there is an area behind the pharmacy counter for prescription medication and medical supplies such as syringes. Retail pharmacies may also carry many treatment supplies:

- A variety of sports braces for the elbow, wrist, knee, ankle, lower back, and ribs.
- Ace® bandages for wrapping sprained body parts.
- Varied sizes of gauze to cover burns and cuts.
- BAND-AIDS® for minor cuts and scrapes.
- A variety of thermometers to monitor temperature.
- Sphygmomanometers for monitoring blood pressure.
- Supplies for diabetics, such as blood glucose monitoring devices, lancets, and Chemstrips®.
- Supplies to relieve eye irritation, such as Visine® and saline solution.
- Contact lens care products, such as cleaning solutions, wetting agents, and protective cases.
- Sun screens with variable UV ratings to help prevent skin cancer.

Additionally, retail pharmacies stock a wide variety of over-the-counter (OTC) medications:

- Medication for arthritis, such as Zostrix® and JointRitis®.
- Medication for diarrhea and gas, such as Imodium AD® and Gas-X®.
- Medication for dry, itchy skin, such as Gold Bond® and Cortaid®.
- Medication for lice, such as Nix® and Rid®.
- Medication for hemorrhoids, such as Tucks® and Preparation H®.
- Medication for constipation, such as Ducolax® and Fleet's® enemas.
- Medication for muscle relief, such as BenGay® and Capsicum.
- Medication for jock itch, such as Cruex®.
- Medication for nausea, such as Emetrol® and Nauzene®.
- Medication for allergy relief, such as Bronkaid® and Primatene®.
- Medicated creams for muscle and joint pain, such as Flexall® and Sportscreme®.
- Sleep aids, such as Unisom® and Sominex®.
- Analgesics (pain relievers), such as Excedrin® and Percogesic®.

This is only a sampling of the products offered in a typical retail pharmacy. There are many different brands and varieties. It is important that pharmacy clerks become familiar with the different products in order to better serve their customers.

Stocking Shelves in the Hospital Pharmacy

Hospital pharmacies are designed to provide medications for inpatients. As a result, they carry different types of stock than retail pharmacies. Although the hospital pharmacy may carry OTC products, they are not displayed for customer purchase. OTCs in the hospital pharmacy will often be mixed in with the bulk prescription drug items.

unit dose: a package of medication that contains a single dose.

Many hospitals use the **unit dose** system of dispensing oral medications (Figure 6-2). In this system, each dose of the medication is packaged separately. Opening one container does not affect any of the other doses. This helps to reduce cross-contamination between drugs. It also reduces the chance of medication errors, since each drug dose is labeled with the complete name and strength of the medication. The medication is clearly identifiable right up until the time the nurse administers the dose to the patient.

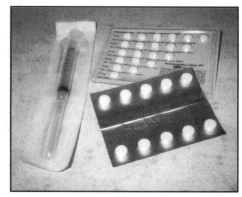

Figure 6-2: Many medications are packaged in unit doses.

Most hospital pharmacies purchase their medications already packaged in unit dose containers. Some drugs, however, are not available in unit dose packages. The pharmacy may buy those medications in bulk containers and package them into unit doses within the pharmacy. Figure 6-3 shows an example of one type of unit dose packaging equipment.

Hospital pharmacies also carry a much larger supply of injectable drugs than a retail pharmacy. Because hospitalized patients are sicker than those treated by outpatient pharmacies, hospital pharmacies carry a broader inventory of antibiotics, antineoplastics, and emergency medications, many of which are available only for injection.

Chapter Six • Inventory Control in the Pharmacy

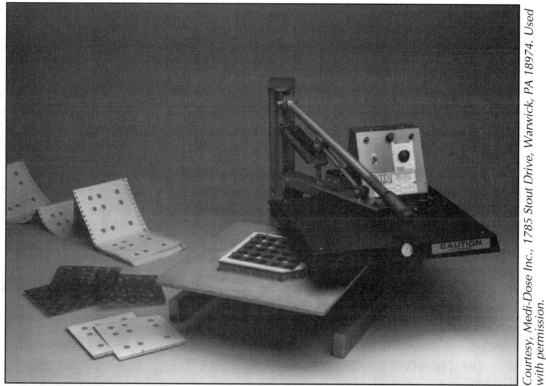

Figure 6-3: This machine seals single sheets of medication.

In addition to the shelves of oral and injectable medications, hospital pharmacies contain an area for storing intravenous (IV) solutions. This is usually adjacent to a separate enclosed room, called a "clean room," where the IV products will be mixed. In the clean room, the IV mixtures are prepared in laminar flow hoods, which sterilize the air inside the hood. This minimizes the risk of contamination when nutrients or other drugs (called **additives**) are mixed into the IV solutions. The pharmacist or technician preparing the **admixtures** must also use **aseptic technique** to avoid contaminating these sterile products.

IV solutions come in a variety of sizes. Solutions for continuous infusion usually come in one liter containers. Intermittent doses of antibiotics may be provided in an **IV piggyback**. IV piggybacks are named for their administration method: they are "piggybacked" into the existing main IV line and run for a brief period of time. When they are empty, the piggyback containers are removed from the main IV line and discarded. Most IV piggybacks contain 50 to 100 mL of fluid in small bags or bottles, although some piggybacks are as large as 250 mL.

aseptic technique: a method of preparing intravenous admixtures to avoid contaminating these sterile products.

IV piggyback: a small IV bag containing medications that is set up to intermittently infuse in conjunction with a larger IV bag.

Many IVs have a short shelf life, so the admixtures are prepared as the patient needs them. This also cuts down on waste, since critically ill patients often have changes in their medication orders. As a result, the clean room in the hospital pharmacy may operate 24 hours a day, 7 days a week.

Stocking Shelves in the Home Infusion Pharmacy

Home infusion pharmacies are like hospital pharmacies in that they carry large amounts of injectable drugs and IV solutions. However, home infusion pharmacies may not use piggybacks for intermittent infusion. Instead, each home infusion pharmacy will carry a variety of specialized delivery devices, such as the CADD® pumps and Intermate® systems.

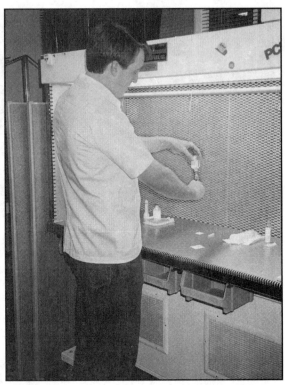

Figure 6-4: A Pharmacy Technician Preparing Intravenous Solutions

Drug Distribution in a Hospital Pharmacy

Drug distribution for inpatients begins with an order written on the patient's chart. These orders look different from a standard prescription because they do not include all of the prescriber's preprinted information. However, the abbreviations and symbols used to interpret **chart orders** are the same as those used on prescriptions.

chart orders: the prescriber's instructions for nursing care, diet, treatments, laboratory tests, and medications for an inpatient.

Pharmacy clerks working in a hospital may be responsible for making hourly rounds to the nursing stations to pick up copies of the chart orders that have been written. These copies may be photocopies, handwritten transcriptions, or direct copies using NCR (no carbon required) physician order forms. Transmitting the chart orders to the pharmacy can also be done electronically, through the use of FAX machines or the hospital computer system. Many hospital pharmacies discourage the use of telephone orders because of the risk of error.

Chapter Six • Inventory Control in the Pharmacy

Common Intravenous Fluids

Dextrose 5% in water (D_5W)	Provides fluid replacement and calories.
Dextrose 50% as a 50 mL bolus	Used in hypoglycemia to correct low blood sugar.
Sodium chloride 0.9% (NaCl 0.9%) (isotonic)	Normal saline (NS) for fluid replacement. A physiological salt solution. It helps correct low serum sodium.
Sodium chloride 0.45% (½NS)	Fluid and sodium replacement.
Sodium chloride 3% or 5% (hypertonic)	Corrects severe sodium depletion.
Dextrose/saline mixtures (D5 ½NS, D5NS)	Provide fluid, sodium, and calories.
Lactated Ringer's solution (also called Ringer's Lactate)	Balanced electrolyte solution roughly equivalent to electrolyte concentration of potassium, calcium, sodium, and chloride in the plasma.
Lactated Ringer's solution with 5% dextrose (D_5LR)	As above, with added calories.
Ringer's solution	Contains more sodium and chloride than lactated Ringer's solution.
Plasmanate	Plasma expander.
Human serum albumin	Plasma expander.
Dextran	Synthetic plasma expander.
Mannitol	Osmotic diuretic to increase urine output.

Figure 6-5: Commonly Ordered IV Solutions

pharmacy patient profile: a confidential record containing medical and billing information, as well as a list of the medications the patient has received.

Once received in the pharmacy, the medication orders are entered onto a **pharmacy patient profile**. Patient profiles list all of the medications that a patient is to receive, including single doses, STAT medications, routinely scheduled drugs, and PRNs. The profile is continually updated as new medications are ordered and previous medication orders are changed or discontinued. The profile usually includes information about the patient's diagnosis and medical history. Such data provides the pharmacist with adequate information for monitoring the patient's response to drug treatment.

The profile is often computerized, allowing access to the patient's medication information throughout the hospital. Nurses may use a version of the profile as their Medication Administration Record (MAR) (Figure 6-7). The MAR is the legal record of all the doses that a patient has received. It becomes part of the patient's chart and may also be used for billing the patient.

Unit Dose Distribution

In a unit dose system, patient medications are generally distributed in cassettes or cubicles (Figure 6-6). Each patient has his or her own cassette drawer, labeled with the patient's name, medical record number, and room number. Cassettes fit into a carrier, which is then loaded into the nurse's medication cart (Figure 6-8). The medication cart can be locked to protect the drugs from theft or tampering.

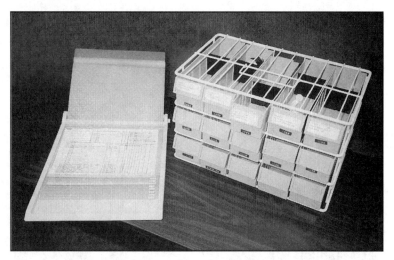

Figure 6-6: Unit doses of medications are stocked in patient drawers for each shift. The cabinets are then placed in the medication cart.

Chapter Six • Inventory Control in the Pharmacy

ABC MEDICAL CENTER 1234 Medical Plaza Drive Anytown, US 01234 (123) 555-1234		PATIENT'S NAME: JOHN SMITH ROOM #: 6033			
NURSE'S SIGNATURE/TITLE	**INITIALS**	**ALLERGIES:** PENICILLIN			
Sally Marshall, RN	SM				
Jack Kea, RN	JK				
Thomas Johes, LPN	TJ				

Continuing Medication Record

Order Date	Stop Date	Medication/Dosage/ Route/ Frequency	Time	Date/ Initials			
				5/14	5/15	5/16	5/17
5/14 JK		Digoxin 0.25mg PO QD Hold if pulse < 60	9	JK P.72	SM P.70	SM P.70	
5/14 JK	5/18 @ 24	Prednisone 5mg PO q8h x 5 days	8 16 24	JK SM TJ	SM TJ JK	SM TJ JK	

One-Time/PRN/STAT Medications

Date	Medication/Dose/Route/ Frequency	Time/Initial	Reason	Result
5/15	Ibuprofen 400mg PO q4h PRN	9:30 AM SM	Leg Pain	10:30 AM relief from pain

Figure 6-7: A Medication Administration Record (MAR) on a Patient's Chart

The pharmacy personnel may fill the cassettes every 24 hours, or as often as once each shift, depending on the hospital policy. Cassettes are filled with only those medications that the patient will require during the fill period. As new medications are ordered, the pharmacy provides the nurse with additional unit doses. If a medication order is changed, the pharmacy personnel will exchange the unit doses for the new medication. Oral, injectable, and topical medications can be placed in the cassette drawers. Some injectables are not available in unit-dose; for those drugs, **multi-dose vials** will be dispensed.

multi-dose vial: a container that has several doses of a medication in it.

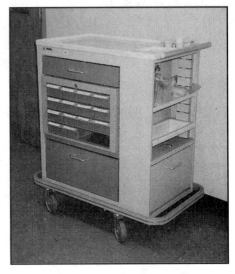

Figure 6-8: A Medication Cart

In the unit dose systems, patients are charged only for the medications that have been taken from the cassette drawer. When the filled cassettes are delivered to the nursing station, they are exchanged for the cassettes that have been used during the previous fill period. The used cassettes are returned to the pharmacy and restocked for the next fill period, using a "fill list" generated from the patient's profile. As the unit doses are added to the cassette, the patient is charged for those doses that are being replaced.

Although cassette filling can become repetitious, accuracy is extremely important. Filling the cassettes requires reading the labels of *each* individual unit dose container. Unit dose containers pulled from the same bin should all be the same drug, but there can be mix-ups in the stock. This usually occurs when someone isn't paying close attention as they return unused drugs to the bins. To avoid harmful errors, each unit dose label must be read very carefully to ensure that it is the right drug, strength, and dosage form for that patient's order. In addition, the correct number of doses for the next fill period must be accurately counted into the cassette. If there aren't enough doses in the cassette, the patient may not get the doses at the correct time. (See Figure 6-10)

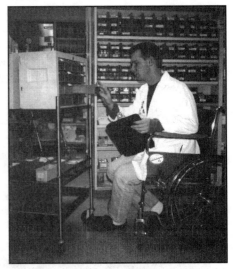

Figure 6-9: Accuracy is essential when filling cassettes.

Robotic systems are playing a role in unit dose drug distribution in some large hospitals. Long robotic arms fill cassettes by pulling bar-coded unit doses from hanging racks. Robotic filling systems are virtually error-free, as long as the medications have been bar-coded correctly. In hospitals that use these systems, the pharmacy staff keeps the hanging racks filled with properly coded unit dose medications.

Hospital policy determines whether controlled substances are distributed in unit dose cassettes. Some hospitals prefer to dispense controlled substances as ward stock, so that they can be kept in a central location. This makes it easier for the nurses to count the controlled substances each shift and to keep a perpetual inventory of the doses used. The central location for controlled substance storage may be a double-locked drawer in the medication cart, or it may be a locked cabinet within the nursing station.

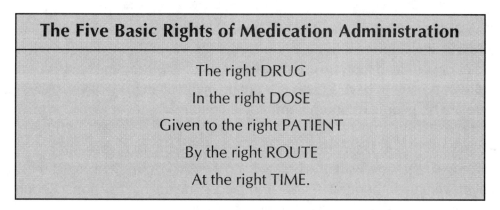

Figure 6-10: The Five Basic Rights of Medication Administration

Automated Dispensing Systems

Many large hospitals are now using automated dispensing machines, such as the Pyxis® system, for their inpatient medication distribution. These machines are on the patient wards, usually near the nursing station. The machines look like cabinets with a computer terminal on top and locked drawers underneath. The drawers contain a variety of drugs that might be needed for patients on that ward.

In hospitals using this type of automation, pharmacy staff stock the dispensing machines with unit doses of drugs instead of putting them into individual patient cassettes. To obtain a specific dose, the nurse must first access the patient's medication profile on the computer. The computer then unlocks the correct drawer, allowing only that drug to be retrieved from the cabinet. Bar codes are sometimes used to guarantee that the nurse selects exactly the right medication.

These systems automatically record the dose of medication used and charge the patient for the drug. This also alerts the pharmacy that the medication needs to be replaced. Much of the repetition of cassette filling is eliminated by these systems.

Transporting Medication

Transporting Medication in a Hospital Pharmacy

Pharmacy clerks in a hospital will be responsible for pushing or carrying medications in specially-made containers. These containers are generally made of steel, aluminum, or heavy plastic. They may be small enough to hold with one hand. Some large carts may require pushing.

When transporting the containers, good **body mechanics** are essential. For example, it is important to push the cart while maintaining the cart within 20 inches of your lead foot. **Overextension** may lead to straining back muscles. It is also important to have a clear view of the hallway in front of you. Make sure there are no people or equipment blocking your way.

When you have to leave the cart unattended, be sure to push it out of the way and leave it against a wall. It is best to keep the cart within sight at all times. This will prevent unauthorized people from accessing the medications. Report any suspicious people to the hospital security force.

Transporting Medications from a Retail or Home Infusion Pharmacy

When the pharmacy clerk is requested to transport medication to people in their homes, it is very important to practice safety at all times. Map out your route before getting in the car. Call customers and get directions if necessary or use the Internet to print out maps and directions. Make sure that your supervisor knows your route. It is a good idea to make sure that others know where you are going and when they can expect you back.

During the time you are a student, you probably will not be allowed to make deliveries in the community. Be sure to check with your instructor before accepting an assignment like this.

Because deliveries are made in cars, standard driver safety precautions should always be used. This includes the use of a seat belt. Many states require drivers and passengers to use seat belts. Even if your state does not require safety belts, the pharmacy's insurance may require that drivers of company vehicles use them. Be sure to check on your pharmacy's policy.

In addition to seat belt use and defensive driving, you will need to take extra care when driving through neighborhoods. Keep your eyes open for suspicious people or circumstances. Stay in well-lighted, open areas. If an area does not look safe, do not stop. Get direction from your supervisor on what to do when you do not feel safe.

Keep the car doors locked at all times, especially when coming to a stop and every time you leave the car. Go directly to the door of the house, apartment complex, or business; do not hesitate or stop to talk with bystanders. As you approach the residence or business, watch for people who are standing around in groups or who act suspicious in any way. Ask to speak directly with the person who has ordered the medication. Be alert and businesslike, and project an attitude of professionalism. Do not allow anything or anyone to distract you from your delivery.

Once you have identified the person to receive the medication, collect the money and keep yourself in sight of others. It is generally not a good idea to stay and speak with customers, although you may find you will be asked into the home. Store all the money as you have been directed by your supervisor. You will generally be given directions to keep money out of sight. Make sure the money is not left in a visible location in your car.

Keep some kind of log of your deliveries, even if not required by your employer. You can use the information to keep track of your time and deliveries. If questions arise, you will be able to refer to your own notes to help answer any questions from customers or fellow employees.

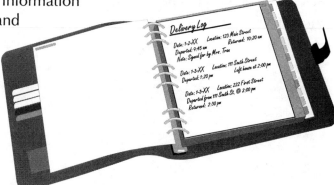

Figure 6-11: Keep a log of your deliveries.

Once you have returned to the pharmacy, have someone assist you in accounting for the money, charge slips, or checks collected. This should be done immediately upon returning; delays leave room for errors. Your accuracy in accounting for medications and money collected will impress your employer.

Chapter Summary

To provide good customer service and patient care, pharmacies must have adequate supplies of medications. Inventory control is the process of maintaining the medication supply by ordering, stocking, and keeping track of the products that are bought and sold by the pharmacy.

Hospital and retail pharmacies stock different types of medications, because their customers and patients have different needs. Regardless of the type of medication, attention must be paid to the shelf life of the products and their proper storage. Improper storage might cause a medication to lose its potency before its expected expiration date. This can result in a significant dollar loss for the pharmacy.

Medications are ordered and distributed differently in a hospital pharmacy than in a retail pharmacy. Because hospitals often use unit dose or automated distribution systems, the drug stock may be purchased in single-unit packages, rather than bulk bottles. Hospital pharmacies may buy medications in bulk containers and then package them into unit-doses.

The pharmacy clerk plays an important role in inventory control by assisting the pharmacist and technician in purchasing, storage, and delivery of drug products. Understanding the inventory control process is essential to your success.

Chapter Six • Inventory Control in the Pharmacy 6-19

Name _____
Date _____

Student Enrichment Activities

Circle T for True, or F for False.

1. T F   Pharmacies keep specific dosage forms together to quickly locate and fill a specific prescription.

2. T F   Unit dose refers to a system of dispensing in which each dose of medication is packaged and labeled separately.

3. T F   Drugs never lose their potency before the expiration date.

4. T F   Retail pharmacies stock shelves for customer's convenience and ease in finding high demand or high profit items.

5. T F   A pharmacy patient profile refers to the nurse's assessment of the patient's condition.

6. T F   Pain medication is commonly administered via an IV piggyback.

7. T F   An NDC number is a unique numeric identifier of a specific drug product.

8. T F   Medication orders may be transmitted to the pharmacy via computers or paper copies of physician orders.

9. T F   Even if the state law that doesn't require a driver to wear a seat belt when driving, most insurance companies do.

10. T F   Syringes in a retail pharmacy are placed on shelves along with all other over-the-counter items.

Complete the following statements.

11. A multi-dose vial contains _____ _____ of a medication.

12. Items stocked in a retail pharmacy, other than prescriptions, could include _____ medications, _____, and health and beauty aids.

13. A _____ is used to store the patient's medications inside the medication cart.

14. Medications can be purchased _____ from the manufacturer or through a pharmacy _____, which stocks drugs from many companies.

15. When delivering medication to a customer's home, precautions that the pharmacy clerk should take include:
    A. _____
    B. _____
    C. _____
    D. _____

Chapter Seven
Staying Healthy in the Workplace

Objectives

After completing this chapter you should be able to do the following:

1. Define and correctly spell each of the key terms.
2. Explain ways to promote optimal physical health.
3. List potential health hazards for pharmacy clerks.

Key Terms

- aerobic exercise
- biohazardous substances
- hypertension
- preventive healthcare
- range of motion (ROM)
- wellness

Introduction

Work in the pharmacy requires the ability to stand for long periods of time. It also involves bending down and lifting medications and supplies. Although this type of work can be demanding, advance planning eases the workload. This chapter will present information on how to minimize work-related physical and mental stress, and achieve what medical professionals call **wellness**.

wellness: the state of optimum health.

Maintaining Good Health

Working in the healthcare industry means exposure to a number of physical and mental stresses. The single most important strategy for successfully meeting those pressures is to be in good physical health. The medical community puts great emphasis on **preventive healthcare**, focusing on proper eating habits, weight control, stress management, exercise, cholesterol reduction, and smoking cessation. In the core textbook of this series, *Introduction to Clinical Allied Healthcare*, Chapter Nineteen has a thorough discussion of healthful living.

preventive healthcare: healthcare that focuses on patient education to promote health and prevent disease.

Control Your Weight

People who are overweight are at a higher risk for a number of health conditions: joint and bone problems (arthritis and pain), adult-onset diabetes, asthma, cardiovascular diseases, varicose veins, hypertension, myocardial infarctions, depression, low self-esteem, and strokes. Opinions vary on the best method for determining a healthy weight. In fact, most experts agree body composition is a much more useful guideline than weight in determining a person's level of fitness. Body composition refers to the amounts of water, fat tissue, and lean tissue that make up a person's total body weight. It is measured as a ratio between an individual's lean body mass and fat and is often referred to as a person's percentage (%) of body fat. For instance, two men could each weigh 200 lbs. One of the men could be considered physically fit, while the other might be considered overweight. It all depends on the person's body composition. However, determining and monitoring an individual's body composition requires the assistance of trained personnel and ongoing reassessment. So, many people still rely on various height and weight charts for guidance in determining if they are at a healthy weight.

Even with height and weight charts, there is much disagreement over which is the best one to use. Some tables consider frame size, age, and gender, while others do not. Furthermore, none of the tables distinguish excess fat from muscle. This means that a person with a lot of muscle may appear to be obese when, in fact, he is not. Body Mass Index (BMI) has been the medical standard for obesity measurement since the early 1980s. Government researchers developed it to take height into account in weight measurement. However, many of the same problems that exist with the height and weight tables apply to BMIs as well. Although the term *obese* often carries a negative connotation in normal usage, in the field of healthcare it is a non-judgmental term that simply indicates a body mass index within a certain range.

The Body Mass Index information on the next two pages is from the U.S. Government Report, *Nutrition and Your Health: Dietary Guidelines for Americans, Fifth Edition (2000)*. This information may be useful in determining if you are at a healthy weight.

Adults may follow the directions below to evaluate their Body Mass Index (BMI). It is important to note that not all adults who have a BMI in the range labeled "healthy" are at their most healthy weight. For example, some people may have lots of fat and little muscle. A BMI above the healthy range is less healthy for most people; but it may be fine if you have lots of muscle and little fat. The further your BMI is above the healthy range, the higher the weight-related risk (see Figure 7-1) for health problems. If your BMI is above the healthy range, you may benefit from weight loss, especially if you have other health risk factors.

How to Evaluate Your Weight (Adults)

1. *Weigh yourself and have your height measured. Find your BMI category in Figure 7-1. The higher your BMI category, the greater the risk for health problems.*

2. *Measure around your waist, just above your hip bones, while standing. Health risks increase as waist measurement increases, particularly if waist is greater than 35 inches for women or 40 inches for men. Excess abdominal fat may place you at greater risk of health problems, even if your BMI is about right.*

3. *How many other risk factors do you have?*

   - *Do you have a personal or family history of heart disease?*
   - *Are you a male older than 45 years or a postmenopausal female?*
   - *Do you smoke cigarettes?*
   - *Do you have a sedentary lifestyle?*
   - *Has your doctor told you that you have high blood pressure?*
   - *Do you have abnormal blood lipids (high LDL cholesterol, low HDL cholesterol, high triglycerides)?*
   - *Do you have diabetes?*

The higher your BMI and waist measurement, and the more risk factors you have, the more you are likely to benefit from weight loss.

NOTE: Weight loss is usually not advisable for pregnant women.

BMIs slightly below the healthy range may still be healthy unless they result from illness. If your BMI is below the healthy range, you may have increased risk of menstrual irregularity, infertility, and osteoporosis. If you lose weight suddenly or for unknown reasons, see a health care provider. Unexplained weight loss may be an early clue to a health problem.

Keep track of your weight and your waist measurement, and take action if either of them increases. If your BMI is greater than 25, or even if it is in the "healthy" range, at least try to avoid further weight gain. If your waist measurement increases, you are probably gaining fat. If so, take steps to eat fewer calories and become more active.

ARE YOU AT A HEALTHY WEIGHT?

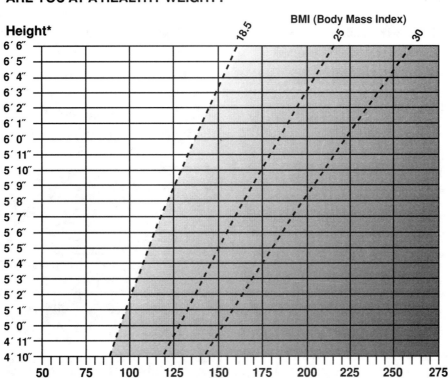

BMI measures weight in relation to height. The BMI ranges shown above are for adults. They are not exact ranges of healthy and unhealthy weights. However, they show that health risk increases at higher levels of overweight and obesity. Even within the healthy BMI range, weight gains can carry health risks for adults.

Directions: Find your weight on the bottom of the graph. Go straight up from that point until you come to the line that matches your height. Then look to find your weight group.

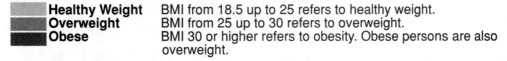

Healthy Weight BMI from 18.5 up to 25 refers to healthy weight.
Overweight BMI from 25 up to 30 refers to overweight.
Obese BMI 30 or higher refers to obesity. Obese persons are also overweight.

Source: Report of the Dietary Guidelines Advisory Committee on the Dietary Guidelines for Americans, 2000, page 3.

Figure 7-1: Suggested Weights for Adults, Ages 25 to 29

Source: Nutrition and Your Health: Dietary Guidelines for Americans, Fifth Edition (2000). http://www.health.gov/dietaryguidelines. March 2001.

Get Plenty of Exercise

Being in good physical condition also means to exercise regularly and to refrain from smoking. A standard exercise program should include at least 20 minutes of **aerobic exercise** three times a week. There are many references available in your local bookstore on the subjects of diet, exercise, and psychological well-being. Many of them can give you information on a thorough health promotion plan. Consult your doctor about the best exercise program for you.

aerobic exercise: exercise designed to make the heart and lungs work harder, causing an increase in oxygen intake and use.

If you find you are unable to work a full exercise program into your schedule, consider the following suggestions. You could pack a healthy lunch and combine a light lunch with a walk. This will improve your physical health, assist with weight control, and enhance your ability to handle the pressures of your job. In addition to taking a lunch, be sure to take your breaks. Sometimes walking outside for some fresh air will help to improve your attitude. Take your breaks out of your work area. A little distance from the hectic pace of the pharmacy will enhance your productivity.

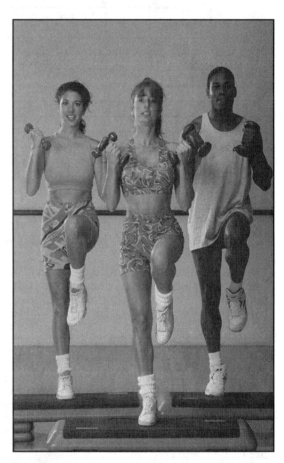

Figure 7-2: Some activities burn more calories than others.

You can also exercise at your desk. Be sure to practice the following simple **range of motion (ROM)** exercises throughout the day:

range of motion (ROM): the maximum range through which a joint can move.

- Shoulder rolls: To relax neck muscles, perform one shoulder roll at a time or both at the same time. Rotate your shoulders forward and then backward for 10 to 20 times.

- Head rolls: To relax your shoulders, roll your head in a full circle clockwise and then counterclockwise several times.

- Walking: If you are sitting or standing at a desk or computer terminal, walk around at regular intervals.

You can plan your work so that the amount of sitting, standing, and bending is paced throughout the day. If you are not accustomed to standing for long periods of time, you will find this difficult at first. Train yourself to vary your body position to ease the transition to the physical demands of the job.

Get Plenty of Sleep

Sleep deprivation can result in inattentiveness on the job. Accidents can occur when your mind is not rested. Adequate sleep can also prevent a person from getting ill by keeping the body's immune system from becoming run down. People are much more likely to become ill when they are sleep-deprived.

Avoid Hypertension

Hypertension, also called high blood pressure, is known as the *silent killer* because it often does not exhibit any signs or symptoms to the patient until it has reached a dangerous level. Untreated, hypertension can lead to a stroke, or heart and kidney damage.

Hypertension can be controlled by reducing the intake of salt, managing stress, exercising, maintaining an acceptable weight, and eating a healthy diet. Sometimes medication may also be necessary.

Signs of high blood pressure, although not always present, can include waking up with a headache over a period of 3 days or more, blurred vision, and general weakness. Do not ignore any of these symptoms. Have your blood pressure monitored regularly.

hypertension: high blood pressure that has been diagnosed on the basis of several random readings of 140/90 or higher; known as the silent killer.

Manage Stress

Stress is present in everyone's life, and especially on the job in a healthcare setting. The American Academy of Family Physicians estimates that symptoms linked to stress are related to about 66% of all visits to a family physician.

Stress is generally defined as the perception that events or circumstances have challenged, or exceeded, an individual's ability to cope. Too much stress can lead to hypertension, chest pain, shortness of breath, headaches, **insomnia**, mood swings, and even a heart attack. Coping with stress is a very individual thing; some people cope much better with stress than others.

There are a number of ways to reduce and relieve stress. Seminars are available in most communities to help individuals cope with today's stressful lifestyles. There are also many books on the subject. The following guidelines can be effective in managing stress.

1. Eat a healthy diet. Some studies have shown that a high intake of the B vitamins can help people cope with increased stress.

2. Develop and maintain a regular exercise program.

3. Know your limits and learn coping mechanisms for stress.

4. Take vacations.

5. Take time for activities that you find restful and stress-free.

Work-related stress can be reduced by planning in advance. To ensure that you arrive to work on time and stress-free, you might take steps to reduce your morning routine: lay out your clothes for the next day before you go to bed at night, make your lunch ahead of time, or set the alarm for a half hour earlier. Once you are at work, prepare your work space by making sure you have the supplies (pens, papers, and so on) to do the job. Preparation makes a big difference in the work flow.

If you identify a problem in the workplace, speak with your supervisor to resolve the situation before additional stress develops. Pick a time that is not busy and prepare in advance by having some suggestions for improving the situation.

Avoid the Inappropriate Use of Alcohol and Drugs

Many drugs, including alcohol, taken in excessive amounts can result in addiction— and possibly death. People often cope with high levels of stress by using drugs. However, drugs do not eliminate the problem that caused the stress in the first place. Drugs are simply an escape. In fact, prolonged drug usage simply makes matters worse by creating the potential for addiction—thereby complicating the original problem of unresolved stress.

Companionship and healthy activities are great substitutes for drugs. If you feel you are becoming an addict, there are many chemical dependency programs available. Organizations such as Alcoholics Anonymous and Narcotics Anonymous have had great success in helping people overcome addiction. These organizations can be accessed over the Internet at **http://www.aa.org** and **http://www.na.org** respectively.

Workplace Safety

As with most professions, pharmacy work has a few inherent risks. These risks can take the form of **biohazardous substances**, environmental hazards, robberies, and psychological hazards. The psychological hazards have already been noted. A discussion of other common risks follows.

biohazardous substances: preparations that can damage living cells; examples include cancer chemotherapy drugs and radioactive medications.

Biohazardous Substances in the Pharmacy

Potentially biohazardous substances are used in the treatment of cancers, among other things. These medications may need to be handled with special gloves. The pharmacist will dispense these drugs and mark their containers, usually plastic bags or lead-lined containers. Notify the pharmacist if these medications are spilled or contaminated by other means. If your skin comes in direct contact with these substances, follow your institution's policy regarding clean-up.

Health Tips for Computer Users

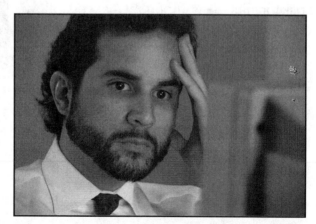

Figure 7-3: Working in front of a computer screen for extended periods of time can cause eye strain.

Eye strain is an environmental work-related hazard. If you are working on a computer terminal, also called a video display terminal (VDT), move away from the screen at regular intervals. You should focus your eyes on objects at varying distances from where you are sitting. This allows your eye muscles to avoid being overstrained by long periods of focusing at the same object. Looking away every 15 minutes or so will reduce the strain on your eyes and neck muscles.

As you work on the computer throughout the day, rest your hands frequently. Remember that when using a keyboard, your wrists should remain as straight as possible; that is your wrists should not be flexed or hyperextended. Repetitive use of your hands can lead to muscle soreness and other complications. Consult with your doctor if you experience numbness, tingling, or pain in your fingers.

Chairs used at computer stations should also be designed for maximum comfort and safety for the employee. Although pharmacy clerks rarely get an opportunity to sit down while on the job, appropriate seating arrangements should be made for those times when sitting is either possible or necessary. For instance, chairs should be a comfortable height so that the user's feet rest flat on the floor, while the VDT monitor is positioned at eye level.

Preventing Sprains and Strains

Hospital workers are recognized as one of the leading groups of employees with sprain and strain injuries. Within this group, the employees who work directly with patients experience more strains and sprains than those who do not provide direct patient care. However, pushing, pulling, and stocking shelves in the pharmacy can present a risk for injury. It is important that you follow the principles of good **body mechanics**. Hospitals routinely conduct classes on how to lift, bend, and stoop properly. Be sure to attend these classes at regular intervals. Although you may be tempted to skip such a class, you must remember that you are responsible for maintaining your health, and such classes can help you accomplish this task.

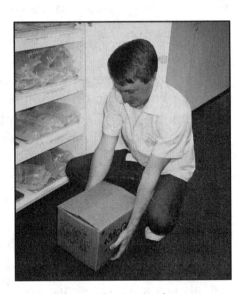

Figure 7-4: The use of proper body mechanics can prevent injuries when lifting heavy objects.

As discussed in Chapter Six, be sure to push carts and not pull them. Keep them within 20 inches of your body. Overextending yourself when pushing carts can lead to low back injuries. Ensure that the load you are pushing is well within your physical capability. Ask for assistance when necessary.

Avoiding Falls

Falls occur for a variety of reasons. Some causes are beyond the control of the victim. The best protection against falls is to wear sturdy shoes with nonskid soles. In addition, take time to look for potential hazards. Use extra caution when walking on a wet floor or in construction or remodeling areas. Use care when going around corners in high traffic areas of the workplace. As with defensive driving, an awareness of potential hazards is your best defense against injury.

Robberies

Robberies are becoming an increasing problem in pharmacies. Every institution promotes the policy that human life is more important than the drugs and/or money being stolen. As advised earlier, do not make yourself a hero by trying to stop a robbery. Do as you are told. Do not try to communicate in code to other employees. Follow your institution's guidelines on how to act in a pharmacy robbery. If your employer does not hold robbery drills, suggest these drills as a precaution.

Chapter Summary

Being a pharmacy clerk involves certain risks, both mental and physical. Pharmacies can be stressful places to work. For example, you may be standing for long periods of time, which requires stamina, or you may be bending and lifting cases of medications, which increases your risk of sprains and strains. Additional stresses may include eyestrain resulting from prolonged computer use and risk of exposure to hazardous substances due to improper use or storage of such materials.

You can minimize these risks by preparing in advance. Become aware of the specific risks you face in the workplace and develop strategies to avoid injury and stress. Learn to recognize your body's signs of stress and find ways to relieve and/or manage that stress before it becomes a problem. By watching your diet and getting plenty of exercise, you can relieve stress and reduce your risk for health problems such as hypertension, bone and joint disorders, depression, myocardial infarctions, strokes, and more. To avoid workplace injuries, always practice proper body mechanics.

Including these health-promoting strategies in your daily routine is a gift you give yourself. Maintaining your own wellness will enable you to help others achieve their optimum health.

Chapter Seven • Staying Healthy in the Workplace   7-13

Name _____
Date _____

Student Enrichment Activities

Complete the following exercises.

1. Use a separate sheet of paper to design your own personal exercise plan.

2. Use a separate sheet of paper to explain how you can minimize the risk of eye strain while working on the computer.

3. Describe two exercises to relax your shoulder and neck muscles.
   A. _____
      _____
   B. _____
      _____

4. List three ways you can minimize work-related stress.
   A. _____
   B. _____
   C. _____

Fill in the blanks.

5. Untreated, _____ can lead to a stroke, or heart and kidney damage.

6. Aerobic exercises are designed to make the _____ and _____ work harder, causing an increase in _____ intake and use.

7. It is important to follow the principles of good _____ _____ to reduce the risk of sprains and strains.

8. In the event of a robbery, do not attempt to be a _____.

Circle T for True, or F for False. (Not graded; however false answers may warrant consideration by the respondent.)

9. T F I am at my ideal body weight.

10. T F I eat a healthy, well-balanced diet.

11. T F I am now involved in an exercise program that is realistic to my current fitness level and available time.

12. T F My blood pressure is normal.

13. T F I get enough sleep most nights.

14. T F I do not overindulge in alcohol.

15. T F I do not take recreational drugs.

16. T F I handle stress well.

17. T F I take vacations.

Glossary

A

*accounting: a system of record keeping that tracks business transactions, such as money owed by customers and money spent for operating costs.
*accounts payable: money owed by a business to creditors such as suppliers or other businesses.
*accounts receivable: money owed by a customer or other debtor on a current debt.
accreditation: acknowledgment that an organization, institution, or facility, such as a pharmacy, has met established committee standards.
additives: medications and certain nutrients, particularly those added to IV solutions.
admixtures: products (usually intravenous solutions) that contain one or more added drugs or nutrients.
*adverse drug reactions: unfavorable and undesirable effects or toxicity in response to a pharmacological substance.
*aerobic exercise: exercise designed to make the heart and lungs work harder, causing an increase in oxygen intake and use.
*aerosol: a substance suspended in a pressurized gas and administered as a mist, such as asthma medication or throat sprays.
agitation: excessive restlessness.
allergic reaction: an excessive sensitivity to a chemical substance. Symptoms may include rash, facial swelling, or difficulty breathing.
antagonistic: working against, or blocking, an action.
*apothecary and avoirdupois systems: rarely used systems of weights and measures that use specific ratios of grains, ounces, minims, quarts, and pounds.
*aseptic technique: a method of preparing intravenous admixtures to avoid contaminating these sterile products.
assignment of benefits: payment of benefits made directly to the provider rather than to the patient.

B

*back-ordered: temporarily unavailable from the supplier. Also referred to as "short."
beyond-use date: expiration date; the date after which a patient should not use a medication, because its stability and potency cannot be guaranteed.
*bioavailability: the rate and extent of absorption of a drug into the bloodstream.
*biohazardous substances: preparations that can damage living cells; examples include cancer chemotherapy drugs and radioactive medications.
body mechanics: the efficient and safe use of the body during activity.

C

capitation: a financial arrangement where a certain amount of money is received or paid out based on membership in the plan rather than on services rendered.
capsule: an oral solid dosage form that contains a drug within a gelatin shell.
***certification:** demonstration of knowledge and abilities.
***chart orders:** the prescriber's instructions for nursing care, diet, treatments, laboratory tests, and medications for an inpatient.
***chemical name:** a drug name consisting of a formula that describes its chemical composition.
chemotherapy: the use of drugs or chemicals to treat or control diseases such as cancer.
chewable: designed to be chewed; a type of soft, flavored tablet that is chewed into small pieces before being swallowed.
***clinic:** a center, often a separate department in a hospital, that treats individuals who are patients, but have not been admitted to the hospital.
***compliance:** taking a medication accurately, according to its directions for use.
***confidential:** private; not to be discussed with others.
***controlled substances:** drugs defined and regulated by *The Controlled Substances Act of 1970*, including narcotics, hallucinogens, depressants, and stimulants.
***Controlled Substances Act of 1970:** a law enacted to control the distribution and use of drugs with the potential for abuse, such as narcotics (opiates and opium derivatives), hallucinogens, stimulants, and depressants.
***copayment:** the share of medical costs for which the insured patient is responsible.
***coverage:** the amount and extent of financial responsibility. (ie, an insurance company may pay for a medication, but it will only pay for a specified dollar amount or a certain percentage).
***CPhT:** certified pharmacy technician; one who has passed the national PTCB exam.
cream: a semi-solid topical dosage form that readily disperses in water.
***cross-contamination:** the making of a clean object or person unclean by contact with another object or person.
***customer service:** courteous assistance provided to a customer as determined by his or her needs.

D

DEA: abbreviation for Drug Enforcement Administration.
deductible: an amount that must be paid by the patient or customer before the insurance company will pay any benefits. There are usually individual deductible amounts and a total amount for the family that must be met.
dependents: the individuals who are covered by an insurance policy through another person. (Usually a spouse and children.)
disenrollment: the process of terminating insurance coverage.

*dispense: to provide medication as prescribed by a physician or other qualified person.
diversion: redirecting the delivery to someone other than to the intended facility or patient.
dosage forms: pharmaceutical products (tablets, lotions, suppositories, etc.) designed to deliver a drug to the patient by a specific route of administration.
*drug: a chemical substance used to diagnose, prevent, or treat disease.
*Drug Enforcement Administration (DEA): an agency of the federal government responsible for regulating the import and export of narcotics and other substances, the transport of such drugs across state lines, and drug trafficking.
drug utilization review (DUR): checking the appropriateness of each prescription against the patient's allergies, medical history, and other medications.

E

effervescent: designed to rapidly dissolve with the release of gas bubbles when placed in water (for example, Alka-Seltzer).
*eligibility: satisfaction of all of an insurance company's requirements to become qualified to receive insurance benefits.
*elixir: an oral dosage form prepared by combining one or more drugs with a mixture of water, alcohol, sweeteners, and flavors.
*emulsion: a combination of two liquids that, though mixed, will not dissolve into one another (ie, oil and water).
EPO: exclusive provider organization; similar to an HMO, but called exclusive because patients must stay within the network to receive the benefits of the plan.
*expiration date: the date after which the stability and potency of a drug cannot be guaranteed; also called the beyond-use date.

F

FDA: abbreviation for Food and Drug Administration.
*formulary: a list of drugs for which an insurance company has agreed to provide partial or total reimbursement; a list of drugs that a hospital commonly stocks.
*fraudulent: unauthorized, false, forged.

G

gatekeeper: the term given to the primary care physician who must authorize care to be given by other providers except in real emergencies. A common requirement of HMOs.
*generic equivalent: a drug with the same chemical structure and bioavailability as a trade name product.
*generic name: the nonproprietary name of a drug, under which the drug is licensed and which is used by every manufacturer of that drug.

genetic engineering: the process of creating new genetically coded cells through the introduction of chromosomes from another species.
gum: a dosage form that contains a drug in a chewable base.

H

healthcare provider: the physician, facility, or supplier that provides a medical service.
HMO: health maintenance organization; a healthcare plan that provides care to enrolled members for a predetermined amount of money, usually prepaid on a per-member monthly basis. However, because of the increase in self-insured businesses and contracts with different financial arrangements, not all HMO plans require prepayment. Most utilize primary care physicians as gatekeepers, require preauthorization, and offer a limited panel of providers. Not all assume total financial risk so that some risk for medical expenses may be assumed by the providers.
***hygiene:** cleanliness.
***hypertension:** high blood pressure that has been diagnosed on the basis of several random readings of 140/90 or higher; known as the silent killer.

I

idiosyncratic reaction: describes an individual reaction to a drug caused by genetics or other factors specific to that person; in some cases, this reaction may be opposite of the drug's expected action.
***ineligible:** in a pharmacy, a term used to describe a person who is not allowed or not qualified to receive insurance benefits.
***injectable:** generally describes medications that can be administered by using a needle.
inpatient pharmacies: facilities that provide medication and pharmaceutical care to patients receiving treatment in a hospital.
insomnia: chronic difficulty sleeping.
insurance: a contract made between two people or two groups of people, in which one agrees to provide certain specified health benefits to the other.
***insured:** an individual whose medical costs are covered, in part or wholly, by specific arrangements with an insurance company; the individual who holds the policy.
***interdependence:** actions or activities that require one person to work with another.
intradermal: refers to injections given into the skin, such as in tuberculin or allergy testing.
intramuscularly: in the pharmacy, it refers to medication that is injected into the muscle by way of a needle and a syringe.
intravenous (IV): directly into the vein.
***intravenous solutions (IVs):** sterile fluids that are injected directly into a vein. These solutions may contain medications, nutrients, or supplements that aid in the body's normal functioning.

IPA: independent practice association; an organization that contracts first with a managed care plan and then with individual providers who agree to provide services at a reduced rate either by capitation or fee-for-service.

*IV piggyback: a small IV bag containing medication that is set up to intermittently infuse in conjunction with a larger IV bag.

L

lotion: a topical drug suspension.
*lozenge: solid medication administered by dissolving in the mouth.

M

MCP: managed care plan; any system of healthcare management that incorporates ways to control costs through methods such as gatekeepers, preauthorization, panels of contracted providers, etc. Examples include HMO, IPA, PPO, and POS plans.
Medicaid/Medi-Cal: state provided health insurance for economically depressed individuals and families. Coverage is usually very specific and limited.
Medicare: federal insurance provided to people over the age of 65, those who have permanent kidney failure, and people with certain disabilities. This is the fastest growing group of insured people. Coverage usually is very specific.
*metric system: a uniform system of measurement that uses the meter, gram, and liter as the units of measurement, based on units of ten.
*multi-dose vial: a container that has several doses of a medication in it.

N

*narcotic: a drug that suppresses the central nervous system to relieve pain; can be habit-forming.
NDC: abbreviation for National Drug Code.
*NDC number: a unique number that identifies each drug product. The NDC number indicates the name of the manufacturer and the name, strength, dosage form, and package size of the drug product.

O

ointment: a semi-solid topical dosage form that repels water.
ophthalmic: pertaining to the eye.
*oral: refers to the mouth. In the pharmacy, it refers to medication given by mouth.
otic: pertaining to the ear.
*outpatient: a patient who receives treatment from a healthcare facility without being admitted to a hospital.

outpatient pharmacies: facilities that provide medication and pharmaceutical care to patients who do not require hospital care; includes clinic pharmacies, chain drug stores, and other retail pharmacies.
overextension: extension beyond normal range of motion.
***over-the-counter (OTC):** refers to nonprescription medications that can be purchased in most drugstores and some supermarkets.

P

package inserts: leaflets, which are attached to or included with medication bottles, that provide the extended labeling information required by the FDA.
patent: a document that grants an exclusive right to produce or sell a product.
PCP: primary care physician; a physician who serves as gatekeeper for a managed care plan. Usually a family practitioner, internist, pediatrician, or obstetrician/gynecologist who sees the patient first and then makes decisions as to whether to authorize care by other providers.
***perpetual inventory:** an on-going system of tracking drugs received in the pharmacy and sold by the pharmacy.
***pharmaceutical care:** services that improve a patient's health through the appropriate use of medications.
***pharmacist:** someone who is trained and licensed to evaluate medication use, prepare and dispense medications, and provide counseling and drug information to patients and healthcare workers.
***pharmacokinetics:** the manner and rate by which the body absorbs, distributes, metabolizes, and eliminates a drug. Often referred to as "kinetics."
***pharmacology:** the study of drugs and their actions.
***pharmacy:** the department in a hospital, clinic, or a store in the community that dispenses medication.
***pharmacy clerk:** an allied health worker who works in a pharmacy assisting the pharmacist and customers.
***pharmacy patient profile:** a confidential record containing medical and billing information, as well as a list of the medications the patient has received.
***pharmacy technician:** an allied health worker with advanced on-the-job training and/or education, who assists the pharmacist and customers (training and education requirements vary among the states).
PharmD: the Doctor of Pharmacy degree awarded to pharmacists upon completion of their college education; requires a minimum of six years of college coursework.
physician's assistant (PA): a healthcare professional with specialized training who is directed and overseen by a physician and who can perform certain physician duties.
POS: point of service; an arrangement where patients may receive care outside of their plan, but will receive reduced benefits and will have to pay more out of pocket.
powder: a solid substance that has been ground into small particles.

Appendix A • Glossary

PPO: preferred provider organization; a plan in which patients can receive services from providers of their choice, but receive higher benefits if they go to providers contracted with the plan.
prescribers: healthcare providers who are legally entitled to order prescription medications.
*prescription: (often called a script) an order to dispense a medication that specifies the drug, dosage, frequency, and amount of medication to be given. It also provides information about the prescriber and the patient.
*preventive healthcare: healthcare that focuses on patient education to promote health and prevent disease.
PTCB: abbreviation for the Pharmacy Technician Certification Board.

R

*range of motion (ROM): the maximum range through which a joint can move.
rapidly-disintegrating: describes a type of tablet that quickly dissolves in the patient's saliva and which can be taken without water.
rehabilitation: the restoration of a patient or a part of the body to maximum function following an illness or injury.
*reimbursable: in a pharmacy, medications for which the patient's insurance company has agreed to provide payment.
replicated: reproduced; produced in the same form as the original.
*retail pharmacy: a facility that supplies prescription and nonprescription medication to customers in a particular community. It can be located in a drugstore, medical building, or grocery store, or it can be a freestanding building.
route of administration: the method of delivering the drug to the patient's body. Includes oral, injectable, topical, rectal, etc.
RPh: registered pharmacist; any pharmacist who is legally entitled to practice pharmacy by virtue of passing a licensing examination and meeting state requirements.

S

Schedule I drug: controlled substance having no legal medicinal use in this country.
Schedule II drug: controlled substance that is the most highly addictive and do have current medical use.
Schedule III drug: controlled substance that has the potential to be addictive, but are not considered as addictive as Schedule II drugs.
Schedule IV drug: controlled substance that has a tendency to be addictive and are frequently used abusively, but less so than Schedule II or Schedule III drugs.
Schedule V drug: controlled substance that has the least potential for drug abuse because of the small amount of narcotics contained in the drug.

sensitivity: an excessive response to the usual dose of a drug, causing exaggerated effects.
sharps: needles or other sharp devices that can puncture the skin and which have the potential to transmit blood-borne diseases.
***sharps container:** a plastic container, usually red, that is designed for the safe disposal of used sharps.
***shelf life:** the length of time a product can be kept in stock before its contents are altered by age.
***side effect:** unintended reaction, such as headaches or nausea, resulting from the use of a medication.
solution: a liquid dosage form in which the drug is completely dissolved.
***STAT:** Now! This order or request must be handled immediately.
***strength:** the amount of drug contained in each tablet, capsule, or teaspoonful of a medication. For liquids, this is sometimes called the *concentration*.
subcutaneous: beneath or introduced beneath the skin.
sublingual: under the tongue.
***sundries:** various small items often sold in a pharmacy, such as safety pins, bandages, sunglasses, etc.
***suppository:** semi-solid medication administered by melting or dissolving in the rectum, vagina, or urethra.
suspension: a liquid dosage form in which a drug powder floats and settles. Must be shaken well before use.
synergistic: a reaction produced when one substance enhances or adds to the effects of another substance; a reaction produced from the combined effects of two or more agents acting together.
synthesis: produced in a lab by the reaction or combination of chemical ingredients.
syrup: a sugar and water solution, which may be flavored. When used as a dosage form, a syrup contains one or more dissolved drugs.

T

tablet: an oral dosage form made by compressing powders into a solid cake.
therapeutic effect: the desired response to a drug.
***third-party payor:** someone other than the patient who pays for prescription medications; third parties are usually government programs, insurance companies, or managed care plans, such as HMOs and PPOs.
titrate: to use more or less of a substance to achieve a desired result.
tolerance: resistance to a drug, such that increased doses are needed to produce the desired therapeutic effect.
***topical:** refers to the surface of the body. In the pharmacy, it refers to the application of medications to the surface of the body.

*trade name: a drug name created by its manufacturer, (ie Coumadin®, or Tylenol®) that may be protected by a trademark; a brand name.
transdermal patch: a small, thin adhesive disk that contains a layer of drug, which is slowly absorbed into the bloodstream when the patch is worn by the patient.

U

*unit dose: a package of medication that contains a single dose.
Universal Claim Form (UCF): a paper form similar to a credit form. Used for manual processing of insurance claims when on-line claims processing (adjudication) is not possible.

V

*vendor: a company that sells a drug. This may be the manufacturer or a wholesaler.

W

*warning/auxiliary label: an additional label attached to a patient's prescription bottle, giving directions regarding the use or storage of the medication, or announcing potentially harmful effects of the medication.
*wellness: the state of optimum health.

* denotes key term

Appendix A-10

Appendix B-1

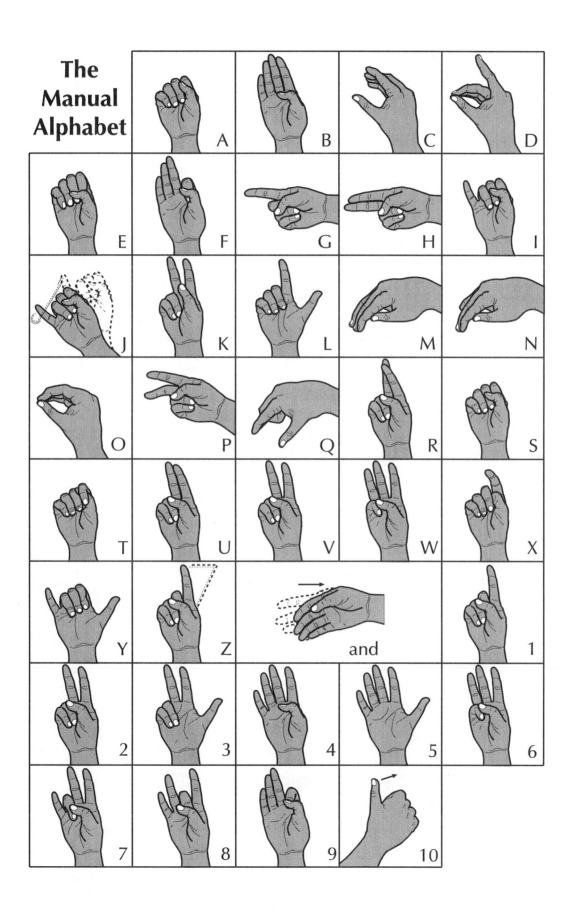

Appendix B-2

Bibliography

Billups, Norman F. and Shirley M. Billups, *American Drug Index, 45th Edition.* Facts and Comparisons, a Wolters Kluwer Company. St. Louis, MO, 2001.

California Board of Pharmacy. *Pharmacy Law with Rules and Regulations, Year 2000, California Edition.* Lawtech Publishing Company. San Clemente, CA, 2000.

Griffith, H. Winter, MD. *Complete Guide to Prescription and Nonprescription Drugs, 1997 Edition.* Berkley Publishing Group. New York, 1997.

Grogan, F. James, PharmD. *The Pharmacist's Prescription.* Rawson Associates. New York, 1987.

Heller, Michelle, and Drebs, Connie. *Delmar's Clinical Handbook for Health Care Professionals.* Albany, NY. International Thomson Publishing Company, 1997.

Lance, Leonard L. and Charles Lacy, Lora L. Armstrong, Morton P. Goldman, *Drug Information Handbook for the Allied Health Professional, 7th Edition.* Lexi-Comp, Inc. Hudson, OH, 2000.

Medical Economics Company, Inc. *Physicians' Desk Reference, 54th Edition.* Medical Ecomonics Company, Inc. Montvale, NJ, 2000.

O'Toole, Marie T., ed. *Miller-Keane Encyclopedia and Dictionary of Medicine, Nursing, and Allied Health, Sixth Edition.* Philadelphia. W.B. Saunders, 1997.

Woolf, Henry Bosley, ed. *Merriam Webster's Collegiate Dictionary, 10th Edition.* G. & C. Merriam Company. Springfield, MA, 1993.

Additional Sources

California Board of Pharmacy, www.pharmacy.ca.gov

U.S. Departments of Health and Human Services and Agriculture, *Dietary Guidelines for Americans, 2000,* www.health.gov/dietaryguidelines/

Appendix C-2

Appendix D-1

Index

A

abbreviations 5-2, 5-6, 5-7
   accuracy 5-6
   dosage forms 4-13
   dosing intervals 5-7
   errors 5-6
   measurements 5-10
   miscellaneous 5-11
   mistakes 5-6
   penmanship 5-6
   roman numerals 5-9
   routes of administration 4-9
accounting
   defined 2-10
accounts receivable
   defined 2-10
acid pump inhibitors 4-26
administration
   medication
      five basic rights 6-15
   routes 4-9
adverse drug reactions 4-17, 4-18
aerobic exercise 7-6
   defined 7-6
aerosols 4-14
   defined 4-14
age 4-15
agitation 4-30
alcohol
   inappropriate use 7-8
Alcoholics Anonymous 7-8
allergic reactions 4-17
   anaphylactic shock 4-17
   breathing trouble 4-17
   rash 4-17
   swelling 4-17
allergic rhinitis 4-27
allergy 4-31
alpha-one blockers 4-23
alpha-two agonists 4-24
American Association of Colleges of Pharmacy (AACP) 1-13
   Internet address 1-13
American Association of Pharmacy Technicians (AAPT) 1-13
   Internet address 1-13

American Drug Index (ADI) 4-19, 6-5
American Hospital Formulary Service (AHFS®) Drug Information 4-19
analgesics 4-28
   combinations of narcotic with non-narcotic analgesics 4-29
   narcotic agonist analgesics 4-28
   non-narcotic analgesics 4-28
anaphylactic shock 4-17
androgens 4-26
anesthetics 4-29
   general 4-29
   local 4-29
angina 4-25
angiotensin converting enzyme (ACE) inhibitors 4-23
angiotensin receptor blockers (ARBs) 4-23
answering the telephone 3-2 thru 3-4
antacids 4-25
antagonistic effect 4-16
anti-anxiety drugs 4-30
anti-emetics 4-25
anti-epileptics 4-29
antiarrhythmics 4-23
antibiotics 4-21
anticoagulants 4-23
anticonvulsants 4-29
antidepressants 4-29
antidiabetics 4-26
antidiarrheals 4-25
antiflatulents 4-25
antifungals 4-21
antihistamines 4-31
antihyperlipidemics 4-24
antihypertensives 4-23
   alpha-one blockers 4-23
   alpha-two agonists 4-24
   angiotensin converting enzyme (ACE) inhibitors 4-23
   angiotensin receptor blockers (ARBs) 4-23
   beta-blockers 4-23
   calcium channel blockers 4-24
antimicrobials (anti-infectives) 4-21
   antibiotics 4-21
   antifungals 4-21
   antiseptics 4-22
   antivirals 4-22

antineoplastics   4-22, 4-27, 6-5
antipsychotics   4-30
antisecretory drugs   4-26
antiseptics   4-22
antispasmodics   4-25
antitussives   4-31
antivirals   4-22
anxiety   4-30
anxiolytics   4-30
apothecary   5-8
apothecary system   5-7
 defined   5-7
approval   4-3
approximate measurement Equivalents   5-11
arthritis   4-27
aseptic technique
 defined   6-9
assistants
 aide   1-3
 legal restrictions   1-3
 pharmacy clerk   1-3
asthma   4-27, 4-32
asthma prevention   4-32
asthma prophylaxis   4-32
attention deficit disorder   4-30
automated dispensing systems   6-15
 bar codes   6-15
avoiding cross-contamination   3-26
avoirdupois system   5-7
 defined   5-7

B

back-ordered
 defined   6-3
back-ordered medications   6-4
bar codes   6-4, 6-15
basic rights of medication administration   6-15
beta-blockers   4-23
beyond-use date   5-12, 6-2
bioavailability
 defined   4-3
biohazardous substances   7-9
 defined   7-9
biotechnology   1-2
bladder relaxants   4-32, 4-33
blood clotting   4-23
blood flow   4-24
blood pressure   4-24, 4-32
blood thinners   4-23
body composition   4-15, 7-2

body mass index (BMI)   7-3, 7-4
body mechanics   6-16, 7-10
body weight   4-15
bone density   4-28
brand name. *See also* drug: trade name.
bronchodilators   4-32
business machines   3-11
 cash register   3-11, 3-13
 credit card scanner   3-13, 3-14
business managers   2-10, 2-11
 responsibilities   2-10

C

calcium channel blockers   4-24
caplet   4-10
capsules   4-10
 elastic shell   4-10
 hard shell   4-10
 liqui-gels   4-10
 liquid gelcaps   4-10
cardiotonics   4-24
cardiovascular system medications   4-23
 antiarrhythmics   4-23
 anticoagulants   4-23
 antihyperlipidemics   4-24
 antihypertensives   4-23
 blood thinners   4-23
 cardiotonics   4-24
 vasodilators   4-24
 vasopressors   4-24
cash register   3-11, 3-13
cassette filling   6-12, 6-14
 accuracy   6-14
central refill pharmacies   1-12
certification
 defined   2-6
 pharmacy technicians   2-6
Chapter Summary   1-14, 2-14, 3-30, 4-33, 5-19, 6-18, 7-11
characteristics
 pharmacy personnel   1-4, 1-6
chart orders   6-10
checks   3-16
chemical name
 defined   4-4
chewable tablets   4-11
cholesterol   4-24
clean room   6-9
cleaning
 work surfaces   3-28

cleanliness
  gloves   3-26
  handwashing   3-26
  handwashing technique   3-27, 3-28
  hygiene   3-28
  pharmacy   3-26
clinic
  defined   1-4
clinic pharmacy   3-5
clinical trials   4-3
colds   4-31
combinations of narcotic with non-narcotic analges   4-29
committee assignments   3-30
common systems   5-7
  apothecary system   5-7
  avoirdupois system   5-7
communication   3-9
  effective skills   3-8, 3-9
compliance
  defined   2-4
computer health tips   7-9
computers   1-3, 1-5, 1-12, 2-4, 2-7, 2-9, 3-2, 3-13, 3-21, 3-22, 3-30, 4-16, 4-20, 5-5, 5-11, 5-14, 5-19, 6-10, 7-6, 7-9, 7-10, 7-11
conception prevention   4-28
confidential
  defined   5-14
confidentiality   5-16
  outdated prescriptions   5-15
  patient   5-15
constipation   4-26
contamination of medications   3-29
contraceptives   4-28
controlled substance   4-8
  categories   4-8
controlled substances   4-7, 6-4, 6-5, 6-15
  Controlled Substances Act of 1970   4-7
  defined   3-17
  depressants   4-7
  hallucinogens   4-7
  narcotics   4-7
  Schedule I drugs   4-7
  Schedule II drugs   4-7
  Schedule III drugs   4-7
  Schedule IV drugs   4-8
  Schedule V drugs   4-8
  stimulants   4-7
Controlled Substances Act of 1970   4-7
copayment
  defined   3-17

corticosteroids   4-27
coughs   4-31
counseling   5-14
coverage
  defined   3-19
CPhT
  defined   2-6
creams   4-14
credit card purchases   3-15
credit card scanner   3-13, 3-14
cross-contamination
  avoiding   3-26
  defined   3-26
customer identity   5-13
customer payments   1-3
customer service   1-6, 3-2 thru 3-4, 3-11
  answering the telephone   3-2 thru 3-4
  clinic pharmacy   3-5
    answering the telephone   3-5
  defined   3-2
  expiration date   6-3
  hospital or clinic pharmacy
    answering the telephone   3-4
  hospital pharmacy   3-5
    answering the telephone   3-5
  retail pharmacy
    answering a telephone   3-2
    answering the telephone   3-3
  upset or difficult customers   3-5
customer service requests   1-3
customers
  upset or difficult   3-5

D

DEA number   5-3
decongestants   4-32
defined
  vendors   6-3
delusions   4-30
dentists   2-8
depressants   4-7
depression   4-29
dermatitis   4-27
diabetes   4-26
diagnosis   3-26
diarrhea   4-25
digestive system medications   4-25
  antacids   4-25
  anti-emetics   4-25
  antidiarrheals   4-25

antiflatulents 4-25
antispasmodics 4-25
emetics 4-25
laxatives 4-26
stool softeners 4-26
ulcer treatments 4-26
disease states 4-16
dispense
  defined 1-3
dispensing date 5-12
dispensing ounces 5-9
diuretics 4-32
dosage forms 4-10
  abbreviations 4-13
  injectables 4-15
    intradermal (ID) injections 4-15
    intramuscular (IM) medications 4-15
    intravenous (IV) medications 4-15
    subcutaneous (SC or subQ) medications 4-15
  oral liquids 4-12
    emulsions 4-12
    solutions 4-12
    suspensions 4-12
  oral solids 4-10
    capsules 4-10
    gums 4-12
    lozenges 4-12
    tablets 4-10
  topical 4-13
    powders 4-14
    semi-solid 4-14
    suppositories 4-14
    topical solutions 4-13
    topical suspensions 4-14
    transdermal patches 4-14
dosages 4-15
  age 4-15
  body composition 4-15
  body weight 4-15
  disease states 4-16
  gender 4-16
  sensitivity 4-16
  tolerance 4-16
  toxicity 4-15
dosing intervals 5-7
dress codes 3-28

drug 4-9. *See also* medication.
  administration
    routes 4-9
  approval 4-3
    Food and Drug Administration (FDA) 4-3
  chemical name 4-4
    defined 4-4
  clinical trials 4-3
  defined 4-2
  development 4-3
  dosage forms 4-10
  dosages 4-15
  effects
    adverse drug reactions 4-17
    allergic reactions 4-17
    antagonistic 4-16
    idiosyncratic reaction 4-17
    side effects 4-17
    synergistic 4-16
    therapeutic effect 4-17
  FDA-approved uses 4-18
  generic equivalent 4-3, 4-4, 4-6
  generic name 4-4, 4-5
    defined 4-4
  industry 4-3
  manufacturers 4-3 thru 4-5, 4-20, 5-9
  new 4-3, 4-6
  non-prescription 4-6
  off-label use 4-18
  OTC 4-6
  patent 4-4
  risk versus benefit relationship 4-17
  schedules 4-7, 4-8
  slang names 4-6
  testing 4-3
  trade name 4-4
    defined 4-4
drug classifications 4-6
  controlled substances 4-7
drug development 4-2
drug distribution 6-10
  hospital pharmacy 6-10
  unit dose distribution 6-12
drug effects 4-17
Drug Enforcement Administration (DEA) 4-7
Drug Facts and Comparisons® 4-19
drug overdose 4-25

drug reference materials 4-18
   American Drug Index (ADI) 4-19
   American Hospital Formulary Service (AHFS®)
      Drug Information 4-19
   Drug Facts and Comparisons® 4-19
   Drug Topics® Red Book® 4-19
   package inserts 4-18
   Physician's Desk Reference® (PDR®) 4-19
   United States Pharmacopeia – National Formulary
      (USP-NF®) 4-20
   United States Pharmacopeia Drug Information
      (USP-DI®) 4-20
drug reimbursement 3-17
drug salts 4-5, 4-6
drug suppliers 2-11
Drug Topics® Red Book® 4-19
drug utilization review (DUR)
   defined 2-4
drugs. *See also* medications.
   inappropriate use 7-8

E

ear drops 4-13
edema 4-32
effective communication 3-8
effervescent tablets 4-11
elastic shell capsules 4-10
electrolyte replacements 4-22
electrolytes 4-22
elements of a prescription 5-3
eligibility 3-17, 3-21
   defined 1-9
elixirs 4-12
   defined 4-12
emetics 4-25
employee thefts 5-18
emulsions
   defined 4-12
endocrine (hormone) system medications 4-26
   androgens 4-26
   antidiabetics 4-26
   antineoplastics 4-27
   corticosteroids 4-27
   estrogens 4-27
   osteoporosis treatments 4-28
   progestins 4-27
   thyroid replacements 4-28
enemas 4-13
enlarged prostate treatments 4-33
enteric coating 4-11

estosterone deficiencies 4-26
estrogens 4-27
   contraceptives 4-28
exercise 7-6, 7-8
expectorants 4-32
expiration date 5-12, 6-2, 6-3
   defined 6-2
expired products 6-2
eye drops 4-13
eyewashes 4-13

F

falls 7-11
FDA 4-4, 4-6, 4-18, 4-20. *See also* Food and
   Drug Administration.
   approved uses 4-18
   post-marketing surveillance 4-3
federal crime 5-17, 5-18
fever 4-31
film coated tablets 4-11
five basic rights of medication administration 6-15
flatus 4-25
Food and Drug Administration (FDA) 4-3,
   4-20. *See also* FDA.
   Internet address 4-20
formulary 5-5
   defined 3-21
fractures 4-28
fraudulent
   defined 5-17
fraudulent prescriptions 5-17
   warning signs 5-17
fungus 4-21

G

gas 4-25
gastroesophageal reflux disease (GERD) 4-26
gelcaps 4-11
geltab 4-11
gender 4-16
generic equivalent 4-3, 4-4, 4-6
   defined 4-3
generic medications 4-4
generic name 4-4, 4-5
   defined 4-4
genetic engineering 1-2
gloves 3-26
gums 4-12

H

hallucinations 4-30
hallucinogens 4-7
handwashing 3-26, 4-22
  procedure for 3-27, 3-28
handwashing technique 3-27, 3-28
hard-shell capsules 4-10
hay fever 4-27
headaches 4-30
health
  healthy diet 7-7, 7-8
  healthy weight 7-2
    body mass index (BMI) 7-3, 7-5
    height and weight charts 7-3
    suggested 7-5
  healthy weights
    suggested 7-5
  maintaining good 7-2
  weight control 7-2
heart failure 4-24
heart rhythm 4-23, 4-25
heartburn 4-25, 4-26
height and weight charts 7-3
high blood pressure 4-23
histamine-2 (H-2) antagonists 4-26
HMO 1-2, 1-12, 2-10, 3-17 thru 3-19
home infusion pharmacies 6-10, 6-16
  transporting medication 6-16
hormones 4-27
hospital environment 1-9
hospital pharmacies 1-9, 3-5, 6-8 thru 6-10, 6-16. *See also* inpatient pharmacies.
  chart orders 6-10
  drug distribution
    unit dose distribution 6-12
  key people and concerns 1-10
  medication administration record (MAR) 6-12, 6-13
  pharmacy patient profile 6-12
  transporting medication 6-16
  unit dose distribution 6-12
    robotic systems 6-15
household system 5-7
household units 5-7
hygiene 3-28
  defined 3-26
hypertension 4-23, 4-24, 7-7
  defined 7-7
hypnotics 4-30

I

identification cards 3-21
idiosyncratic reaction 4-17
impotence treatments 4-33
indigestion 4-25
ineligible, defined 3-21
infections 4-21, 4-22
inflammation 4-27, 4-31
inhalants 4-13
injectables 4-15
  defined 4-15
  intradermal (ID) injections 4-15
  intramuscular (IM) medications 4-15
  intravenous (IV) medications 4-15
  multi-dose vials 6-14
  subcutaneous (SC or subQ) medications 4-15
inpatient pharmacies 1-8, 2-12. *See also* hospital pharmacies.
inscription 5-3
insomnia 4-30
insulin 4-26
insurance 3-23, 3-26, 4-6
  carrier 3-26
  companies 4-4
  eligibility 3-21
  identification cards 3-21
  information 5-4
  plans 3-17
    eligibility 3-17
  prior authorization 3-22, 3-23
  terms 3-18 thru 3-20
  third-party plans 3-21, 3-22
  verification 3-22 thru 3-24
Insurance Verification Request 3-24
insured
  defined 3-19
interdependence
  defined 5-2
intradermal (ID) injections 4-15
intramuscular (IM) medications 4-15
intravenous (IV) medications 4-15
intravenous solutions (IVs) 6-9, 6-11
  defined 1-9
inventory control 1-3, 6-1 thru 6-18
  bar codes 6-4
  controlled substances 6-4
    narcotics 6-4
    Schedule II drugs 6-4
  stocking shelves 6-5
IV piggyback, defined 6-9

J

Joint Commission on Accreditation of Health Care Organizations   5-6

L

labels   5-12, 5-13
laxatives   4-26
liqui-gels   4-10
liquid gelcaps   4-10
lotions   4-14
lozenges   4-12
   defined   4-12
lupus   4-27

M

mail order prescription services   1-2
mail-order pharmacies   1-12
malignant tumor cells   4-22
managed care programs
   HMO   1-2, 1-12, 2-10, 3-17 thru 3-19
   Medicare   1-2, 3-20
measurement systems
   apothecary system   5-7
   avoirdupois system   5-7
   converting   5-7
   household system   5-7
measurements   5-7, 5-10
Medicare   1-2, 3-20
medication. *See also* drug.
   categories. *See* Pharmacologic Categories of Medication.
   names   4-5
   routes of administration   4-9
      abbreviations   4-9
medication administration
   five basic rights   6-15
medication administration record (MAR)   6-12, 6-13
medications. *See also* drugs.
   back-ordered   6-4
   beyond-use date   6-2
   commercial packaging   5-9
   contaminated
      disposal   3-29
   contamination   3-29
   expiration date   6-2, 6-3
   expired products   6-2
   manufacturing   1-2, 5-9
   purchasing   6-3
   shelf life   6-2
   sterile products   6-9
   storage conditions   6-5
      freezing   6-3, 6-5
      refrigeration   6-3, 6-5
menopause   4-27
metric system   5-7
   defined   5-8
migraine headaches   4-30
migraine treatments   4-30
mucus   4-32
mucus membranes   4-32
multi-dose vials
   defined   6-14
muscle mass   4-26
muscle spasms   4-25, 4-31
musculoskeletal system medications   4-31
   non-steroidal anti-inflammatory drugs (NSAIDs)   4-31
   skeletal muscle relaxants   4-31

N

narcotic
   defined   3-10
narcotic agonist analgesics   4-28
narcotics   4-7, 4-16, 4-28, 4-29, 5-18, 6-4, 6-5, 7-8
Narcotics Anonymous   7-8
nasal sprays   4-13
nausea   4-25
NDC number
   defined   6-3
needle disposal   3-29
needle stick   3-29
nervous system medications   4-28
   analgesics   4-28
   anesthetics   4-29
   anti-anxiety drugs   4-30
   anti-epileptics   4-29
   anticonvulsants   4-29
   antidepressants   4-29
   antipsychotics   4-30
   anxiolytics   4-30
   hypnotics   4-30
   migraine treatments   4-30
   sedatives   4-30
   stimulants   4-30
new drugs   4-3, 4-6
non-narcotic analgesics   4-28
non-prescription drugs   4-6
non-steroidal anti-inflammatory drugs (NSAIDs)   4-31
NSAIDs. *See* non-steroidal anti-inflammatory drugs

(NSAIDs).
nurse practitioners   2-8
nurses   2-11
Nutrition and Your Health: Dietary Guidelines for Americans   7-3, 7-5

O

office workers   2-11
ointments   4-14
on-line and electronically transmitted orders   6-4
optometrists   2-8
oral
   defined   1-11
oral liquids   4-12
   emulsions   4-12
   solutions   4-12
   suspensions   4-12
oral medications   6-5
oral solids   4-10
   capsules   4-10
   gums   4-12
   lozenges   4-12
   tablets   4-10
organizational structure   2-2, 2-12
   inpatient pharmacy   2-12
   outpatient pharmacy   2-13
osteoporosis treatments   4-28
OTC   2-4, 2-7, 4-8, 6-2 thru 6-4. *See also* non-prescription drugs; over-the-counter.
OTC drugs   4-6, 4-10, 4-17, 4-19, 6-6 thru 6-8
other healthcare workers   2-11
   nurses   2-11
   office workers   2-11
   therapists   2-11
other types of pharmacies   1-12
outdated prescriptions   5-15
outpatient
   defined   3-6
outpatient pharmacies   1-8
outpatient pharmacy   1-11, 2-13
over-the-counter (OTC)   2-4, 6-6, 6-7
   defined   2-4
over-the-counter (OTC) drugs   3-4, 4-6
overactive bladder   4-32
overdosage   4-18

P

package inserts   4-18
pain   4-28
patent   4-3, 4-4

patient
   confidentiality   5-16
      disposal of pharmacy paperwork   5-15
      outdated prescriptions   5-15
   financial records   5-14
patient confidentiality   5-15
patient information
   expiration date   6-3
patient information sheet   5-12
patients   4-17
payments   3-25
   check   3-16
   credit card   3-15
perpetual inventory
   defined   6-4
personnel   2-2
   characteristics   1-4, 1-6
pharmaceutical care
   defined   2-2
pharmacies
   types
      central refill pharmacies   1-12
      hospital (inpatient)   1-9
      mail-order pharmacies   1-12
      other   1-12
      outpatient pharmacies   1-11
      specialty pharmacies   1-12
pharmacists   2-2, 2-5, 4-17
   defined   2-2
   education   2-2, 2-3, 2-4
   licensing   2-3
   responsibilities   2-4
   trust   2-5
pharmacokinetics
   defined   4-5
pharmacologic categories of medication   4-21
   antimicrobials (anti-infectives)   4-21
   antineoplastics   4-22
   cardiovascular system medications   4-23
   digestive dystem medications   4-25
   electrolyte replacements   4-22
   endocrine (hormone) system medications   4-26
   musculoskeletal system medications   4-31
   nervous system medications   4-28
   respiratory medications   4-31
   urinary system medications   4-32
pharmacology
   defined   1-2
pharmacy
   abbreviations   5-2, 5-6, 5-7. *See also* abbreviations.

accuracy 5-6
errors 5-6
mistakes 5-6
penmanship 5-6
assistants
titles 1-3
business machines 3-11, 3-13, 3-14
cleaning
work surfaces 3-28
cleanliness 3-26
dress codes 3-28
gloves 3-26
handwashing 3-26
handwashing technique 3-27, 3-28
hygiene 3-28
defined 1-2
dress codes 3-28
organizational structure 2-2, 2-12
personnel 2-2
characteristics 1-4, 1-6
records 1-3
robberies 5-18, 7-11
schools 2-4
symbols 5-2
technical training 1-7
theft 5-18
types
clinic 1-4
retail pharmacy 1-4
pharmacy clerk
defined 1-3
skills and responsibilities 3-1 thru 3-30
pharmacy clerks
defined 2-7
responsibilities 2-8
state restrictions 2-7
tasks 2-7
technical training 1-7
pharmacy measurements 5-7
approximate measurement equivalents 5-11
common systems
apothecary system 5-7
avoirdupois system 5-7
dispensing ounces 5-9
pharmacy paperwork
disposal 5-15
pharmacy patient profile 3-21
defined 6-12
pharmacy team 2-1 thru 2-14, 5-2. *See also* pharmacy: personnel.
business manager 2-10

drug suppliers and salespeople 2-11
other healthcare workers 2-11
pharmacists 2-2
pharmacy clerks 2-7
pharmacy technicians 2-5
prescribers 2-8
pharmacy technician certification board (PTCB) 2-6
pharmacy technicians 2-5, 2-6
certification 2-6
education 2-5
licensing/registering 2-6
responsibilities 2-5, 2-6
technical training 1-7
training 2-6
PharmD 2-2, 2-3
defined 2-2
physicians 2-8
physician's assistants 2-8
Physician's Desk Reference® (PDR®) 4-19
"pills". *See* tablets. *See also* capsules.
places of employment 1-8
inpatient pharmacies 1-8
outpatient pharmacies 1-8
podiatrists 2-8
poisoning 4-25
post-marketing surveillance 4-3
powders 4-14
prescribers 2-8, 4-5, 4-17, 5-14
defined 2-4
dentists 2-8
license classification 5-3
nurse practitioners 2-8
optometrists 2-8
pharmacists 2-8
physicians 2-8
physician's assistants 2-8
podiatrists 2-8
veterinarians 2-8
prescription 5-1 thru 5-19
beyond-use date 5-12
counseling 5-14
dispensing date 5-12
elements 5-3
inscription 5-3
signatura 5-3
subscription 5-3
superscription 5-3
expiration date 5-12
filling 5-2, 5-4, 5-5
refill authorization 5-14
refill restrictions 5-15

fraudulent 5-17
   processing 5-2, 5-4, 5-5
      refill authorization 5-14
      refill restrictions 5-15
   telephone orders 5-14
prescription blank 5-2
prescription labels 5-7, 5-11
   patient information sheet 5-12
   warning/auxiliary labels 5-12, 5-13
prescription number 5-11
prescription orders
   receiving 2-9
prescription processing 5-4, 5-5, 5-13
prescription transmission 5-3
prescriptions
   defined 1-3
preventive healthcare
   defined 7-2
prior authorization 3-22, 3-23
processing prescriptions 5-5, 5-13
   refill authorization 5-14
product labels 4-5
professional organizations 1-13
progestins 4-27
   contraceptives 4-28
purchasing 6-3
   on-line and electronically transmitted orders 6-4

R

range of motion (ROM) 7-6
   defined 7-6
rapidly-disintegrating tablets 4-11
rash 4-17
receipts 3-26, 5-14
refills 5-14
   authorization 5-14
   requests 5-16
   restrictions 5-15
   telephone requests 5-15
reimbursable
   defined 5-4
reproductive disorders 4-27
respiratory medications 4-31
   antihistamines 4-31
   antitussives 4-31
   asthma prophylaxis 4-32
   bronchodilators 4-32
   decongestants 4-32
   expectorants 4-32
responsibilities and skills 3-1 thru 3-30

restful activities 7-8
retail pharmacy 2-8, 6-6, 6-16
   defined 1-4
   transporting medication 6-16
risks 5-18, 7-8, 7-9, 7-10, 7-11
   needle stick 3-29
robberies 5-18, 7-11
robbery
   rules 5-18
robotic systems 6-15
roman numerals 5-9
routes of administration 4-9
   abbreviations 4-9

S

safety 3-29, 5-6, 5-12, 5-17, 5-18, 6-3
   workplace 7-9
salespeople 2-11
Schedule I drugs 4-7
Schedule II drugs 4-7
Schedule III drugs 4-7
Schedule IV drugs 4-8
Schedule V drugs 4-8
sedatives 4-30
seizures 4-29
semi-solid topical dosage forms 4-14
   creams 4-14
   ointments 4-14
sensation elimination 4-29
sensitivity 4-16
sharps container
   defined 3-29
shelf life 6-2
   defined 6-2
shoplifting 5-18
side effects 4-17
signatura 5-3
skeletal muscle relaxants 4-31
skills and responsibilities 3-1 thru 3-30
skin disorders 4-27
slang names 4-6
sleep 7-7
sleep disorders 4-30
solutions 4-12
   elixirs 4-12
   syrups 4-12
sprains 7-10
STAT
   defined 3-4
state
   restrictions 2-7

state boards of pharmacy   1-3
   Internet addresses   1-13
staying healthy   7-1 thru 7-11
   aerobic exercise   7-6
   alcohol   7-8
   biohazardous substances   7-9
   body mass index (BMI)   7-3 thru 7-5
   body mechanics   7-10
   computer health tips   7-9
   diet   7-8
   drugs   7-8
   exercise   7-6, 7-8
   falls   7-11
   healthy weight   7-2
      body composition   7-2
   height and weight charts   7-3
   hypertension   7-7
   Nutrition and Your Health: Dietary Guidelines for Americans   7-3
   restful activities   7-8
   robberies   7-11
   sleep   7-7
   sprains   7-10
   strains   7-10
   stress   7-8
   stress management   7-7
   vacations   7-8
   weight control   7-2
   workplace safety   7-9
sterile products   6-9
steroids   4-27
stimulants   4-7, 4-30
stocking shelves   6-5
   antineoplastics   6-5
   controlled substances   6-5
   home infusion pharmacy   6-10
   hospital pharmacy   6-8
      injectables   6-8
      intravenous (IV) solutions   6-9
      unit doses for oral medications   6-8
   oral medications   6-5
   retail pharmacy   6-6
   storage conditions   6-5
   topical medications   6-5
stomach acid   4-26
stool softeners   4-26
storage conditions   6-3, 6-5
storing medications
   intravenous (IV) solutions   6-9
strains   7-10
strength, defined   5-3

stress   7-7, 7-8
stress management   7-7
Student Enrichment Activities   1-15, 2-15, 3-31, 4-35, 5-21, 6-19, 7-13
subcutaneous (SC or subQ) medications   4-15
sublingual tablets   4-11
subscription   5-3
sugar-coated tablets   4-11
sundries
   defined   6-3
superscription   5-3
suppositories   4-14
suppository
   defined   4-14
suspensions   4-12
suspicious people   5-17
swelling   4-32
symbols   5-2
synergistic effect   4-16
synthesis   4-2
syrups   4-12

T

tablets   4-10
   caplet   4-10
   chewable   4-11
   effervescent   4-11
   enteric coated   4-11
   film coated   4-11
   gelcaps   4-11
   geltab   4-11
   rapidly-disintegrating   4-11
   sublingual   4-11
   sugar-coated   4-11
technical training   1-7
   pharmacy clerks   1-7
   pharmacy technicians   1-7
telephone calls   1-3
telephone orders   5-14
   refill   5-15
testing   4-3
theft   5-18
   rules   5-18
therapeutic effect   4-17
therapists   2-11
third-party payor
   defined   3-17
third-party payors   5-15
third-party plans   3-21, 3-22
thyroid gland   4-28

thyroid replacements 4-28
tolerance 4-16
topical
   defined 1-11
topical dosage forms 4-13
   powders 4-14
   semi-solid 4-14
   suppositories 4-14
   topical solutions 4-13
   topical suspensions 4-14
   transdermal patches 4-14
topical medications 6-5
topical solutions 4-13
   ear drops 4-13
   enemas 4-13
   eye drops 4-13
   eyewashes 4-13
   inhalants 4-13
   nasal sprays 4-13
   nose drops 4-13
   vaginal douches 4-13
topical suspensions 4-14
   aerosols
      defined 4-14
   lotions 4-14
toxicity 4-15
trade name 4-4
trademark 4-4
tranquilizers 4-30
transdermal patches 4-14
transporting medication 6-16
   home infusion pharmacy 6-16
   hospital pharmacy 6-16
   retail pharmacy 6-16
transporting medications
   body mechanics 6-16
troche. *See* lozenges.
trust 2-5
tumors 4-27
types of pharmacies
   central refill pharmacies 1-12
   mail-order pharmacies 1-12
   other 1-12
   outpatient pharmacy 1-11
   specialty pharmacies 1-12

U

ulcer treatments 4-26
   acid pump inhibitors 4-26
   antisecretory drugs 4-26
   histamine-2 (H-2) antagonists 4-26
ulcers 4-26
unit dose
   defined 6-8
unit dose cassettes
   controlled substances 6-15
unit dose distribution 6-12
   cassette filling 6-12, 6-14
   robotic systems 6-15
United States Pharmacopeia – National Formulary (USP-NF®) 4-20
United States Pharmacopeia Drug Information (USP-DI®) 4-20
urinary system medications 4-32
   bladder relaxants 4-32, 4-33
   diuretics 4-32
   enlarged prostate treatments 4-33
   impotence treatments 4-33

V

vacations 7-8
vaginal douches 4-13
vasodilators 4-24
vasopressors 4-24
vendors 6-3
verification 3-22 thru 3-24
veterinarians 2-8
viruses 4-22
vomiting 4-25

W

warning/auxiliary labels 5-13
   defined 5-12
weight control 7-2
weights
   suggested 7-5
wellness
   defined 7-2
work surfaces 3-28
workplace health 7-1 thru 7-11
workplace safety 7-9
wound care 4-22

Y

yeast 4-21